HIDDEN BIBLE
HEALTH
SECRETS

REGINALD CHERRY, MD

SILOAM

Most CHARISMA HOUSE BOOK GROUP products are available at special quantity discounts for bulk purchase for sales promotions, premiums, fund-raising, and educational needs. For details, write Charisma House Book Group, 600 Rinehart Road, Lake Mary, Florida 32746, or telephone (407) 333-0600.

HIDDEN BIBLE HEALTH SECRETS by Reginald Cherry, MD
Published by Siloam
Charisma Media/Charisma House Book Group
600 Rinehart Road
Lake Mary, Florida 32746
www.charismahouse.com

Cover design by Lisa Rae McClure
Design Director: Justin Evans

Library of Congress Cataloging-in-Publication Data:
Names: Cherry, Reginald B., author.
Title: Hidden Bible health secrets / Reginald Cherry, MD.
Description: Lake Mary, Florida : Siloam, 2017. | Includes bibliographical references and index.
Identifiers: LCCN 2017005192 | ISBN 9781629990958 (trade paper) | ISBN 9781629990965 (ebook)
Subjects: LCSH: Holistic medicine. | Alternative medicine. | Health--Religious aspects--Christianity.
Classification: LCC R733 .C483 2017 | DDC 615.5--dc23
LC record available at https://lccn.loc.gov/2017005192

17 18 19 20 21 — 9 8 7 6 5 4 3 2
Printed in the United States of America

CONTENTS

Appendixes

INTRODUCTION

MANY OF YOU are familiar with God's covenant with us for supernatural healing. But did you know that God's original ideal plan for healing was not in the realm of the supernatural?

Let me show you what I mean. Consider this: God's original plan was that man would never get sick in the first place. This was His plan long before He introduced these supernatural means for people to get healed. I want to show you a fascinating thing in the fifteenth chapter of Exodus. God introduced the Israelites to a concept they were not familiar with—healing!

> He said, "If you diligently listen to the voice of the LORD your God, and do what is right in His sight, and give ear to His commandments, and keep all His statutes, I will not afflict you with any of the diseases with which I have afflicted the Egyptians. For I am the LORD who heals you."
>
> —Exodus 15:26

This is the first time God entered into His healing covenant with man. Do you know what's even more fascinating? Immediately after God introduced Himself as the healer in Exodus, He started giving commandments about what the Israelites were to eat. The very next words that God spoke to Moses were, "Indeed, I will rain bread from heaven for you" (Exod. 16:4). In other words, God reveals Himself as a healing God and then immediately gives instructions about what His people will eat. If God is always going to heal supernaturally, why would He be concerned with what the Israelites ate? I want to show you another interesting scripture:

> You shall serve the LORD your God, and He shall bless your bread and your water, and I will remove sickness from your midst.
>
> —Exodus 23:25

The amazing fact of this text is that God was speaking to a group of people who had no sickness at all. Did you know that? Psalm 105:37

reveals that "He brought them out with silver and gold, and no one among their tribes faltered." Not one Israelite was sick, yet God chose that time to enter us into a healing covenant. Do you know what God is showing us?

God is showing us that His perfect will for our healing is that we never become ill in the first place.

Isn't that an amazing facet of God's will for us? I was amazed when I realized how God had positioned these scriptures revealing His perfect way of healing for mankind. This is an important principle of healing.

When we do what we can do in the natural, which means changing our lifestyle—eating habits and exercise, as well as other things—God will act in the supernatural to provide for our healing. We must keep in mind that there are both natural and supernatural means of healing incorporated into God's healing covenant. We need to understand when and how God moves in the natural and when and how He moves in the supernatural to heal.

Diabetes is an excellent example of why God tied nutrition into His original healing covenant. Let's look at the magnitude of this disease alone.

Diabetes is the next great lifestyle event to affect the United States and the world. Twenty-nine million Americans have the disease, and even more frightening, one quarter of those don't know they have it. One-third of American adults are prediabetic.[1] There were 1.7 million new cases of diabetes in 2012, so it is becoming more of an issue all the time.[2]

Diabetes is a vicious disease that prohibits the body from using its most basic energy supply: glucose. It affects almost every body system, including eyes, the heart, kidneys, lower extremities, and skin. Diabetes launches one of the most devastating attacks of any disease against the human body.

But let's look at the dramatic effect nutrition can have on reversing and preventing diabetes. Here are some foods with direct effects on the disease:

+ Psyllium: Just one tablespoon taken per day lowers an individual's glucose levels 11 percent on average and 20 percent after a meal.[3]

+ Grains (oatmeal, oat bran, etc.): Just two servings per day lowers the risk of diabetes by 33 percent.[4]

- Beans (pintos, navy, etc.): The consumption of beans leads to a slow rise in insulin levels, which leads to lower insulin requirements.

- Onions and garlic: These types of produce contain antidiabetic compounds similar to tolbutamide (a prescription for diabetes). These compounds stimulate insulin production.

God enters a healing covenant with man in Exodus 15:26. He then ties freedom from disease (healing) to what we eat (nutrition) in Exodus 16. The above association with foods and healing related to diabetes illustrates God's healing plan beautifully.

SPIRITUAL SECRETS FOR HEALTH AND HEALING

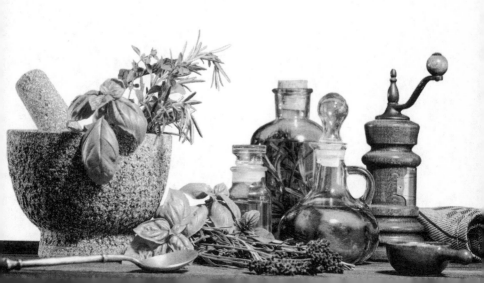

CHAPTER 1

YOUR UNIQUE PATHWAY TO HEALING

Don't be impressed with your own wisdom. Instead, fear the Lord and turn away from evil. Then you will have healing for your body and strength for your bones.

—Proverbs 3:7–8, NLT

So many people in the world today are sick. Virtually none of us will remain untouched by illness, whether it affects our own bodies or the health of those we love. When we are healthy, we give little thought to the way our bodies function, even though that is the time we should be taking steps to maintain our health. Often we wait until we are sick or until some health crisis occurs to make the lifestyle changes necessary to reclaim our health.

You may have picked up this book for a number of reasons. More than likely, you or someone you love is suffering from some illness or disease, and you may be asking yourself, "Does God really want to see me healed?" Or you may already believe that God will heal you, but you may be wondering why He hasn't healed you in a particular way.

Let me answer the question once and for all: *God wants to heal you!* God desires for His people to be healthy and whole, certainly for their own benefit, but also to be able to take His light to a lost and dying world. However, many people seek for their healing to take place in a certain way; most of them prefer it to happen instantaneously, without any real effort on their part.

Perhaps instead of asking, "Why hasn't God healed me this way?," you should ask: "Is there something that I'm doing to hinder my healing? Should I be doing something more than what I am doing now to facilitate my getting well?"

God has a unique pathway for every person, including a pathway to healing. And while I believe in instantaneous healing and I wholeheartedly rejoice when such healing takes place, most of the time God's pathway to healing takes place over a period of time as you walk in obedience to what He tells you to do. Sometimes that involves medical science; other times it incorporates the amazing natural substances that

1

God has placed on His earth for the benefit and healing of His people. New scientific discoveries are taking place all the time that demonstrate that the very substances we need to walk in health exist within nature.

HOW I BECAME A CHRISTIAN DOCTOR

I am a medical doctor who believes in the healing power of God, but that was not always the case. As a young man I was drawn to watch Billy Graham's crusades on television, but that was about the extent of my spirituality. I had always had the desire to help people, and I knew from a very young age that I wanted to be a doctor and do what I could to eliminate sickness and disease from the world.

I attended medical school at one of the most godless institutions I had ever encountered; the people there were not necessarily evil, but they glorified science, reason, and knowledge above all else. Physicians were trained to focus only on the body and perhaps the mind of the patient, but never the spirit—that was left up to the patient's minister or the chaplain on call.

Even so, I was fascinated in medical school with the sheer magnificence of the human body. Now I can express that fascination in the words of Scripture, which declares that we are made "with fear and wonder" (Ps. 139:14). The body has such intricate systems, all working together as a whole; I realized that our bodies are too amazing to have simply evolved on their own from a one-cell organism millions of years ago. There had to be the hand of a Creator involved.

After completing medical school and my internship, I began seeing patients and discovered that they had real problems, many of which had stumped the medical community. There was only so much that doctors knew to do for many of the critical diseases that people faced.

I finally accepted Jesus Christ in 1979 and was born again. Through this life-changing experience I discovered a whole new perspective on this business of making people whole. I began to see that there had to be a source of healing that surpassed what science and medicine had to offer. *Jehovah-Rapha* began to reveal to me that He is the source of all healing, whether it comes by natural or supernatural means. Around this time I was privileged to observe several healings take place that resulted from the direct touch of God. Although I was skeptical at first, when I observed that the symptoms did not return to these persons' lives, I began to understand the power that God has to heal. I realized that He greatly desires to bless His children with healthy bodies and longevity in life.

I grew to accept the truth that God heals today, both naturally and miraculously. And then I began to apply that truth in my medical practice. As I began to seek with my patients the pathway to healing God had designed just for them, I watched people's lives change before my eyes. More and more patients began to walk in health, released from their diseases and free to do what God had called them to do.

God does not want any one of us to suffer needlessly under the curse of disease! It was never His intention for mankind to live under the oppression of sin and the consequences—such as illness—that sin brought into the world. But even after man's fall, God, in His great compassion, made provision for the health of His people. His care for the people of Israel in the Old Testament foreshadows the healing provision He has made for us today.

HEALTH SECRETS OF THE OLD COVENANT

In the Book of Exodus the Lord recorded a wonderful promise for the health of His people. He declared that He would not place "any of the diseases" on His people (Exod. 15:26). We understand that to mean that none of the diseases that plagued the people of that time would enter the camp of the Israelites—that is, as long as they kept the commandments of the Lord. These commandments are timeless; they still hold true for us today. Perhaps one of the greatest secrets the Bible holds for modern man is that the dietary laws of the Old Testament hold great significance for our health and well-being today.

Jesus's death on the cross purchased our healing once and for all, but that does not mean that the dietary laws God had already provided no longer have any meaning. In fact, these ancient Hebrew documents hold fascinating truths about medicine, health, and hygiene that were centuries before their time. Modern medicine continues to prove that the teachings and the health codes given to the Israelites have great value for our health.

God introduced Himself to His people in the Old Testament as *Jehovah-Rapha*, the God who heals. Centuries before Christ died on the cross to purchase our salvation and healing, God was interested in the health of His people! Listen to His promise:

> Worship the LORD your God, and his blessing will be on your food and water. I will take away sickness from among you, and

none will miscarry or be barren in your land. I will give you a
full life span.

—Exodus 23:25–26, niv

God's promise for His people still holds true for us today. But notice
in this passage that He ties the blessings of good health, fertility, and
longevity of life to the blessing that is placed on what they put into
their mouths—their food and water. Some people believe that this verse
means they can simply speak a blessing, or "say grace," over a meal full
of fat, sugar, and carbohydrates, and their health will somehow be protected because the food has been "blessed." But what this promise is
actually telling us is that God has directly tied what we eat and drink to
the maintenance of health in our bodies.

I am convinced that before we receive our healing, we must obey
God's commands as to what we should eat and drink. When we choose
to follow what He tells us to do, we can begin to walk in the health and
blessings He has planned for us. Throughout this book we will explore
some of the health secrets that can be found in the dietary laws of the
Old Testament and learn how they relate to the most common and
destructive ailments that we face in our lives today. Some of these health
secrets include:

+ Prohibitions against fatty foods
+ Prohibitions against eating blood, which has the tendency to
  carry infection
+ Healthy foods that increase longevity and help prevent disease
+ Foods to avoid in order to maintain a healthy lifestyle

Proverbs 3:7–8 tells us, "Don't be impressed with your own wisdom.
Instead, fear the Lord and turn away from evil. Then you will have
healing for your body and strength for your bones" (nlt). In today's culture eating the wrong foods isn't something that we would necessarily call
evil. However, it can bring evil things, such as disease, into our lives. If we
are willing to change our diets and follow God's commands, our health
can be renewed! I encourage you to keep an open mind as we explore the
dietary and health laws God gave to protect His people from disease.

Health Secrets of the New Covenant

In the New Testament God continues to provide healing for His people.
Jesus Christ came to the earth and, through His sacrificial death on the

cross, provided redemption for man, including eternal salvation from sin as well as healing from disease. The prophet Isaiah had foretold this wonderful redemption hundreds of years earlier:

> But he was wounded for our transgressions, he was bruised for our iniquities; the chastisement of our peace was upon him, and by his stripes we are healed.
>
> —ISAIAH 53:5

Throughout His life on the earth, Jesus healed all manner of disease. There are many verses that tell us the magnitude of His healing ministry, such as this one:

> But when Jesus knew it, He withdrew from there. And great crowds followed Him, and He healed them all.
>
> —MATTHEW 12:15

It is important to notice that although Jesus healed multitudes of people, He did so in a variety of ways. There were times when a touch or a word from Jesus healed an infirm person instantly. (See Luke 4:39–40; 6:10.) But not as commonly understood by many people is the fact that sometimes Jesus used *natural substances* through which He caused His healing power to flow.

The most striking example of this method can be found in the Gospel of John, which relates the dramatic healing of a blind man:

> As Jesus passed by, He saw a man blind from birth.... He spat on the ground and made clay with the saliva. He anointed the eyes of the blind man with the clay, and said to him, "Go, wash in the pool of Siloam."...So he went away and washed, and returned seeing.
>
> —JOHN 9:1, 6–7

As these passages indicate, healing can take place instantaneously or as a process that occurs over a period of time. In this case Jesus touched the blind man's eyes as He placed the mud solution on him, but the man was not healed at that time. His healing was complete when he followed Jesus's instructions and washed his eyes in the Pool of Siloam.

So many dear Christians today become disheartened if, after much prayer and petition to the throne of God, they do not receive instant, miraculous healing from their illnesses. But look carefully at what caused this man's healing recorded in John 9. First, he received a touch from Jesus. Then he accepted the application of a natural substance onto the diseased part of his body. And finally, he obeyed Jesus's unique instructions to him as an individual.

This blind man's experience explains for us one of the greatest health secrets of the Bible, one that is often overlooked by well-meaning Christians. I believe it is a vitally important truth that we need to understand in order to walk in the divine health that God would have for us. That truth is this wonderful secret: *God has a unique pathway to healing just for you.*

Let me state it another way: God heals different people in different ways. Some may attend a healing crusade and receive an instant miracle from the Lord. But more commonly God will work through the natural substances that He has provided for us—namely, various foods, vitamins, minerals, and even medications—to work out His healing plan. Sometimes He uses a combination of natural and supernatural methods to effect a cure. The key lies in discovering God's plan for *your own life.* It is not enough to expect what you may have seen occur in the lives of other Christians.

The story of the blind man is in the Bible for a very important reason. There are many other stories of miraculous, instantaneous healings that Jesus performed. But in this story God is challenging us to seek Him for our own pathway to healing. Consider the following important conclusions we can safely draw from the account of the blind man's healing:

+ The blind man wasn't healed when Jesus first touched him.

+ Even so, at the moment of the touch, the healing process had begun.

+ The blind man couldn't necessarily sense the healing process at that time.

+ For the process to continue, the man had to listen to and carefully follow Jesus's instructions to him as an individual.

+ Jesus specifically told him the path to walk on (literally), the name of the pool to which he was to go, and what he was to do when he got there.

As the man was obedient to Jesus's commands, his eyesight was fully restored.

FINDING THE PATH GOD HAS FOR YOU

Wherever I share the gospel and in whatever materials I write, I will always make the hearer and reader aware of what God taught me about the particular pathway to healing He has for each person. God's pathway to healing is available to each of us as we follow His ways and listen to His voice. As you seek healing, I encourage you to pray this prayer:

> *Father,*
>   *I come to You, knowing that You desire to make my body whole. Please show me the path I must take to see the full manifestation of healing in my body.*

Once you have prayed, begin to allow *Jehovah-Rapha* to speak to you and make your pathway to healing clear. Be still before Him and listen. God's Word promises that we can hear His voice, a reality to which many Bible heroes attest. Understand that from the minute you pray this prayer, the process has begun, whether or not you see any immediate change.

Daniel experienced this phenomenon in the Old Testament when he prayed for twenty-one days, crying out to God for an answer on behalf of the people. When the angel of the Lord finally arrived, he told Daniel that from the moment he had begun to pray, the heavenly forces had been set in motion, even though Daniel couldn't see anything taking place in the natural realm. In the supernatural realm, however, the angel had to battle through the opposition to reach Daniel. (See Daniel 10.) So don't give up! Keep praying for your answer. Continue to seek God for His direction, and then when He gives it, be obedient to His commands.

Many times God directs His people to the natural substances that He has already placed within His plant kingdom. Most of the directions that are given throughout this book refer to these amazing natural substances that God gave to man:

> Then God said, "See, I have given you every plant yielding seed which is on the face of all the earth and every tree which has fruit yielding seed. It shall be food for you."
>   —GENESIS 1:29

We are a generation that is different from any other that has walked the face of the earth. Instead of eating food as it naturally comes from the earth, we eat food that our culture has determined has been affected

by herbicides and pesticides of every kind. The air that we breathe is full
of pollutants. We are witnessing the fulfillment of Bible prophecy:

> There will be violent earthquakes, and in various places famines
> and [deadly and devastating] pestilences (plagues, epidemics);
> and there will be terrible sights and great signs from heaven.
> —LUKE 21:11, AMP

But even though these malignant and contagious diseases are virtually surrounding us, God has given our generation the knowledge necessary to extract and concentrate the beneficial elements from the plant
kingdom. Generations before us did not need this divine wisdom as desperately as ours does. As we receive this divine wisdom given to man by
God, perhaps our children and future generations will not suffer the rav-
ages of disease we are experiencing.

DIVINE PURPOSE FOR GOOD HEALTH

Jesus has instructed us to be "the light of the world" (Matt. 5:14). He
told us to "go and make disciples of all the nations, baptizing them in the
name of the Father and of the Son and of the Holy Spirit" (Matt. 28:19,
NIV). But when Christians are sick, fatigued, or just dragging around,
they don't have the strength or energy it takes to be the light of the world
to people who need to know our Savior. They are not interested in going
anywhere to share the good news of the gospel with those who desperately need to hear.

One of the most effective strategies of the enemy is to attack
Christians in their bodies so that they can no longer carry out the work
God has for them. Satan would love to see every one of God's people
lying sick in their beds, focused only on themselves and their own pain
and misery. Let's not allow him to succeed!

Don't just pursue your health so that you can be free of painful
symptoms—seek God's pathway to healing so that you will be able to carry
out His destiny for your life with strength, vigor, and power! Don't allow
the devil to cut your life short with a terminal illness or steal another precious day from your divine destiny simply because you are sick or fatigued.

As you read this book, continue to pray that God will show you what
things He would have you to do to improve your health, perhaps even
using the healing elements that already exist in His natural kingdom. I
encourage you to find your own pathway to healing so that you can carry
His light to a lost and dying world.

CHAPTER 2

DIETARY LAWS FOR TODAY

Do not think that I have come to abolish the Law or the Prophets. I have not come to abolish, but to fulfill.
—MATTHEW 5:17

B UT I'M NOT under the law! I live in grace!"
The burning questions most often asked whenever I share the benefits of following the Old Testament laws for health and hygiene go something like this:

+ "But I'm not under the law! Why should I be concerned with dietary regulations that were established under the Mosaic Law for people living before Christ?"

+ "The Old Testament is outdated and so hard to read. What relevance could it possibly have for my life today?"

+ "Why should I follow the teachings of the Old Testament— especially the ones regarding health and diet? Hasn't Jesus already fulfilled the Law?"

As Christians we have been taught in church that Christ fulfilled the Law, and that is true. Jesus Himself declared, "Do not think that I have come to abolish the Law or the Prophets. I have not come to abolish but to fulfill" (Matt. 5:17). But what does that mean? By virtue of His fulfilling the Law, did He mean it was no longer in effect—that it was abolished? He could not mean that, for that would contradict Jesus's own words. He did not come to abolish the Law or the prophets.

Are the Old Testament laws (recorded in Leviticus and Deuteronomy) no longer valid or useful? That cannot be the case because Jesus said He hadn't abolished or destroyed the Law. There must still be something useful about it, some benefits we will reap for our lives today by keeping the laws of God. Then the question arises: If we decide to keep the Old Testament laws, shouldn't we also keep the sacrificial system, offering burnt offerings to God or having a priest make atonement for our sins? Confusion surrounding God's laws arises because of a lack of understanding them. We need to understand how Jesus fulfilled the Law through His life and through His death.

Because obedience to the Word of God is key to our healing and our health, we need to learn to hear His voice and understand His commands. That begins with searching the words He has already spoken in the Bible, God's written Word.

UNDER THE OLD COVENANT

God gave the Law to His people, the Israelites, first on Mount Sinai with the giving of the Ten Commandments. Later as the Israelites wandered in the wilderness, God set forth, in miniscule detail, all the specific laws that would govern every area of the people's lives.

Today we have trouble relating to all the instructions given to the Israelites to establish their cultural life as a nation. For example, we wonder why God would require His people to purposely and unconditionally burn down any house that showed signs of mildew. Why did He allow people to eat beef but forbid their eating of pork? How could these regulations possibly apply to our lives today?

The fact is that the health and nutritional laws God gave to the Israelites thousands of years ago are some of the most advanced guidelines for avoiding plagues and disease that have ever been developed. Scientific studies are proving that the foods the Israelites were instructed to eat in the Old Testament contain curative properties, or substances that can prevent or even reverse disease. And the "unclean" animals they were forbidden to eat are those that carry the most dangerous bacteria and risk of disease even today. Another example of prohibition to the Israelites was the eating of blood. Now it is common knowledge in the medical community that the blood of animals can carry dangerous infections.

All of this proves that God doesn't just arbitrarily give laws to His people simply to amuse Himself or to prevent us from having a good time—they are always for our own good! It is important to understand that in the Mosaic Law there are three primary categories of regulations:

+ The Ten Commandments, *moral laws*, which govern behavior and relationship with God and one another
+ The sacrificial system, *ceremonial laws*, which govern daily operations of the temple and outline the function of the priests

+ The social hygiene system, *health and dietary laws*, which help God's people prevent disease

Christians today are probably most familiar with the Ten Commandments, the moral laws that were given on the stone tablets to Moses on Mount Sinai. (See Exodus 20.) These moral laws, such as "You shall not murder," are still very much in effect for our lives today (Exod. 20:13). In fact, Jesus took these laws to a new level when He declared that even carrying anger against your brother would put you in danger of judgment the same as murdering him would (Matt. 5:21–22). And with regards to the commandment "Thou shalt not commit adultery," Jesus declared that lusting after a woman was the same as committing adultery with her in your heart (v. 28). We cannot say that because Jesus fulfilled the Law we are free from these moral laws given under the Mosaic covenant.

There is nothing in Scripture that validates the notion that God's health and dietary laws were nullified either. In fact, as I have mentioned, we are beginning to understand the medical significance of these laws as they relate to our own health risks today. Similar to the moral laws, these dietary laws were given for our protection—not for our punishment, as many assume.

Regarding the ceremonial laws that established a priesthood and a system of sacrifice to atone for the sins of the people, they foreshadowed the coming work of Christ on the cross. Of course, because Christ completed—fulfilled—the redemptive work at Calvary, the Scriptures teach us clearly that we have a better sacrifice than that of bulls and goats. We receive by faith the sacrifice of Christ for the forgiveness of our sins. To continue the Mosaic sacrificial system would be to deny salvation through faith in Christ. The writer to the Hebrews states clearly:

> But Christ, when He came as a High Priest of the good things to come, by a greater and more perfect tabernacle, not made with hands, that is to say, not of this creation, neither by the blood of goats and calves, but by His own blood, He entered the Most Holy Place once for all, having obtained eternal redemption. For if the blood of bulls and goats, and the ashes of a heifer, sprinkling the unclean, sanctifies so that the flesh is purified, how much more shall the blood of Christ, who through the eternal Spirit offered Himself without blemish

to God, cleanse your conscience from dead works to serve the
living God?

—HEBREWS 9:11–14

Having stated that the moral laws and the dietary laws that God
gave His people are still in effect, we need to note an important difference between living under the old covenant and life for Christians
under the new covenant. For Israel, the keeping of every single law, in
all three categories—even to the most minute of details—was required
for righteousness. Keeping the Law determined a person's right standing
with God.

Even if an Israelite kept all of the Ten Commandments but slipped up
on a minor detail of the dietary laws, he was considered "unclean" in his
relationship with God and was required to consecrate himself through
various commands to be cleansed because of his sin. (See Leviticus
11:41–45.) His obedience to God's requirements for cleansing was a tan-
gible sign of repentance, which was required under the Law to ensure forgiveness and salvation. It was also necessary to obey God's commands in
order to receive God's promises for health. (See Deuteronomy 7:11–15.)

Because we live under the provisions of the new covenant, we receive
forgiveness for our sins through faith in Christ because of His shed
blood on the cross. Our repentance is expressed through a confession
of faith in the sacrifice of Christ and followed by a surrender to follow
Christ's commands. However, we are not made righteous by our good
works but through faith in Christ, who became our righteousness:

But because of Him you are in Christ Jesus, whom God made
unto us wisdom, righteousness, sanctification, and redemption.

—1 CORINTHIANS 1:30

JESUS FULFILLED THE MOSAIC LAW

When Jesus said He came not to do away with the Law but to fulfill it,
He was validating the laws of the Old Testament. He was giving it His
stamp of approval as the code of behavior by which we should live. Jesus
did not tell us not to keep the moral laws. He raised a higher standard
for the keeping of them.

Did Jesus ever tell us that we no longer need to follow the health and
dietary laws of the Old Testament? No. It surprises many Christians to
learn that Jesus actually kept all of these health laws Himself, and His
disciples did also! As the last Prophet under the old covenant, Jesus kept

all of the laws perfectly, something that no other human being on earth has done or will ever be able to do.

Because Jesus lived a sinless life as the Son of God, He was able to take our sins upon Himself on the cross. As He hung upon the tree and gasped out His final dying breath, His last words were, "It is finished" (John 19:30). He didn't only mean that His life on earth was through— He was declaring that the requirements of the old covenant had been fulfilled. By bearing our sins in His body, Christ had taken the brunt of God's wrath against sin for us.

No longer do we have to keep every single law in order to gain righteousness before God. The apostle Paul declared, "Christ is the end of the law unto righteousness for every one who believes" (Rom. 10:4). Jesus is now our righteousness, and when we place our faith in Him, we gain right standing with God, which establishes a new relationship with our heavenly Father.

Paul described this truth in the Book of Romans when he wrote that it is not by our works that we are saved, but by our faith (Rom. 3:22). It is impossible for anyone to keep all of the old covenant laws perfectly. If it were up to our own abilities, we would surely be lost. But Paul also asked the question, "What shall we say then? Shall we continue in sin that grace may abound?" (Rom. 6:1, NKJV). Since Jesus has already died for us, and because doing good works is not what gets us into heaven, why should we keep the Law at all?

Jesus's work on the cross accomplished our righteousness so that our right standing with God is not contingent on our ability to keep the Law perfectly. However, if we choose to disobey God's laws, we will face consequences from which the Law was given to protect us. Christ's death did not undo the moral laws, making it acceptable to murder someone, tell a lie, commit adultery, or steal. Neither did Christ's death change the composition of "unclean" foods, making it acceptable to eat as many fatty foods as we like, gain twenty extra pounds, or risk damage to our bodies. One explicit New Testament situation affirms some of the dietary laws when outlining proper conduct for Gentile Christians:

> For it seemed good to the Holy Spirit, and to us, to lay upon you no greater burden than these necessary things: that you abstain from things offered to idols, from blood, from things strangled, and from sexual immorality.
>
> —ACTS 15:28–29, NKJV

This passage at least shows that there was no precedent for abolishing the dietary and health laws that had been a part of their lives under the Mosaic Law. The apostle Paul clearly denounced doing anything that would defile our bodies, which have become the temple of God. He declared:

> Know ye not that ye are the temple of God, and that the Spirit of God dwelleth in you? If any man defile the temple of God, him shall God destroy; for the temple of God is holy, which temple ye are.
>
> —1 Corinthians 3:16–17, kjv

The ancient Israelites would never have dreamed of desecrating God's holy temple in their day; how much more should we obediently care for our own bodies in which God Himself dwells?

Blessings and Consequences

If we choose to disobey God's commandments concerning our moral behavior, there are consequences that no believer would question. If Joe murders his neighbor, even if Joe has a change of heart and accepts Christ as his Savior, we still expect him to be sent to prison and face the consequences of his actions. When a person lies, steals, becomes jealous, or otherwise behaves immorally, his actions bring consequences: other people are hurt, lives are ruined, and Satan has a field day for doing what he loves to do—kill, steal, and destroy (John 10:10). Much of the New Testament is dedicated to teaching us how to walk in the love of God through obedience to these commandments. And these same Scriptures teach us there will always be consequences for disobeying God's moral laws.

In much the same way, if you choose to ignore God's laws regarding your diet and your health, you open the door to the enemy to wreak havoc in your life. Though God is not poised, waiting to pour out His wrath on His children when they sin, the fact is that you place yourself in harm's way when you don't eat right or take care of your body properly. While you may not have to sacrifice a sheep or a goat in the temple to restore your relationship with God, there are still unfortunate consequences of your actions:

+ The Spirit of God is grieved. Because the Holy Spirit lives inside of you, He is grieved when you sin or do something to defile the temple of God—your body.

+ You experience a loss of the fruit of the Spirit in your life.

+ You open a door to the works of the enemy. Your failure to eat right may not cause you to lose your salvation, but it certainly can affect your health. The devil would love to take advantage of your poor choices to place sickness and disease on you and your family.

+ You may be unable to fulfill God's destiny for your life and obey His command to be the light of the world. When you are sick in bed or too exhausted to move, you cannot be an effective witness for God.

One mistaken belief some people hold is that sin in a Christian's life somehow directly brings sickness to them, as if sickness were a punishment from God for our sin. What a sad and mistaken belief! It is our own poor choices that bring consequences to our lives in the form of sickness, which Christ died to heal. Though there are instances when choices made by people or generations before us affect us, as in the case of innocent children who suffer disease, we still cannot fault a loving God for that tragedy.

An example of this mistaken belief is seen in the "plague" of AIDS, which some Christians believe was poured out by God to punish homosexuals for their sins. That is simply not true. God never desired that one homosexual—or anyone else—would die of AIDS. It is the behavior patterns that some people choose to practice, violating the laws of God, which place them at risk of disease. Unfortunately many lives have been stolen because of AIDS. Obeying God's law for sexual relations would have prevented the consequences of contracting this dread plague. However, AIDS—or any other disease for that matter—did not come from God.

Jesus declared that He came to reveal the Father to us. His loving nature, reflected in His healing power to the multitudes, is a reflection of the Father's love. Jesus also declared that He came to bring us life and life more abundantly (John 10:10).

I have briefly discussed the relevance for Christians of the Bible's dietary and health laws because many of the Bible's health secrets presented in the chapters of this book have their basis in these laws. I do not believe that Scripture eliminates their relevance for today. And it is a scientific reality that research is confirming their validity for our health and well-being in today's culture. I encourage you to consider making them a part of your life. As you do, I believe you will allow God to pour out His blessings of health and restoration into your body, soul, and spirit.

CHAPTER 3

THE FAITH AND
MEDICINE CONNECTION

*He who does not use his endeavors to heal
himself is brother to him who commits suicide.*

—PROVERBS 18:9, AMPC

C AN I GO to a doctor and still walk in faith?" Many Christians live under the misunderstanding that faith and medicine are separate approaches to healing that contradict one another. It is wonderful to enjoy the fresh revelation in the church today regarding divine healing and faith. God is bringing healing to His people through this understanding of supernatural, instantaneous freedom from disease that is possible through faith.

However, in the midst of this incredible healing move of God there are those among us who haven't received that instant miracle and who begin to wonder, "Why haven't I been healed in this miraculous way?" They may believe they have received a touch from God, sensing His presence in a special way, but the symptoms of their disease remain. They may have even received a supernatural healing, only to discover that the illness has returned a few days or weeks later.

What should these people do? Are they exhibiting a lack of faith if they decide to seek the advice of a physician? Why doesn't God heal them miraculously as He does others? This is a dilemma with which many in the body of Christ grapple. Somehow we have the idea that the correct way for Christians to handle disease is to stand in faith, refuse medicine or other "natural" cures, and wait for a miracle. Divine healing is seen as the better solution to disease. Unfortunately some people are so committed to this viewpoint that they may wait until their deathbed for their miraculous cure, and it still doesn't come. The inevitable results are devastating: a life that could have been lived out in fullness and health is cut short, and faith and trust in God are weakened, both in the patient and in the hearts of those around him or her.

"DO YOU BRUSH YOUR TEETH?"

When people wonder if they should "stand in faith" for their healing rather than seek a natural or medical solution, I like to ask them a very simple question: "Do you brush your teeth?" Of course, we all brush our teeth. But the next questions I ask are more important: "Don't you believe God can heal you of cavities? Can't He prevent plaque buildup and tooth decay from taking place? If so, why do you keep brushing your teeth?"

It's the same reasoning that keeps us from standing in front of a speeding train, raising our arms to heaven, and expecting God to miraculously prevent us from getting hurt. My friends, disease can be heading your way; you may be right in its path. Wouldn't it make sense to do something simple—something natural—to prevent it from hitting you at full force? The Bible tells us:

> He who does not use his endeavors to heal himself is brother to
> him who commits suicide.
> —PROVERBS 18:9, AMPC

I believe this verse can be interpreted to mean that we must do what we know to do to bring healing to our bodies, and then trust God for the rest. There is no validity to the faulty reasoning that concludes our healing must come either from God or from medical intervention. While we must learn to face every situation in faith, we cannot biblically support the claim that walking in faith excludes receiving the natural sources of healing God provided for us on this earth.

THE FIVE P'S OF SPIRITUAL HEALING

There are five basic concepts—the key words of which begin with the letter *p*—that can help people determine what to do, both in the natural and in the spiritual realm, to receive the manifestation of their healing:

1. Understand that Jesus is the Great *Physician*. He is the One to whom you should turn first in times of trouble. He bore stripes on His back that you might be healed (1 Pet. 2:24). Look to Him for your answer.

2. Follow the *peace* of God. Don't pray out of fear or worry. You may not understand what's happening to you in the natural, but you can have God's peace in times of trouble. The

Scriptures teach us to cast our cares upon the Lord (1 Pet. 5:7). The verb tense of this text implies that this is a continual process: cast once, and then keep on casting!

3. Determine God's *pathway* to healing for you. Don't put God in a box or try to manipulate Him into doing what you want Him to do or healing you the way you think He should. If you ask, He will show you His plan for you, which will not be the same one He showed to someone else.

4. Believe in the *power* of healing. When all else fails, stand! Stand in your faith and in your trust in God. Believe that He wants to heal you—that your healing has already been purchased on the cross—without limiting His method for healing you.

5. Pursue your healing with *persistence*. Hang in there. Jesus told parables to emphasize the importance of persevering in prayer, such as the story of the widow who prevailed with the unjust judge (Luke 18:1–8).

GOD'S WAYS ARE NOT OUR WAYS

Why are some people miraculously healed while others are seemingly left to deal with their illnesses "on their own"? At first glance this question seems to call into account the fairness of God. But the truth of the matter is that God loves each of us completely—no more or no less than another—and His desire to heal is unlimited. He is a holy and just God. But He chooses to deal with each of His children in different ways.

One person may indeed receive a miraculous and instantaneous healing from diabetes when prayed for in a healing crusade, while another who is stricken with diabetes may find that the pathway to healing includes diet, exercise, and even medication to keep the diabetes under control. Both persons will experience health and longevity in their lives, but God, in His wisdom, chose different paths for them to take to get to that place of healing.

Earlier in this book I mentioned Jesus healing a blind man by placing a mixture of mud and saliva on the man's eyes and then giving further instructions for the man to go wash in the Pool of Siloam to receive his healing (John 9). However, on another occasion, Jesus healed two blind men by simply touching their eyes and commanding them to see (Matt. 20:29–34). He healed blind Bartimaeus (Mark 10:46–52) by simply saying, "Go your way. Your faith has made you whole" (v. 52).

Now, if we are honest with ourselves, most of us would admit that we would rather be healed the way Bartimaeus was healed. Not only does it seem easier, but also it might give us a more exciting story to tell! The fact is, however, that all four blind men were healed—they could see. The only difference was that the blind man whose story is recorded in John 9 was allowed to participate in the process of his healing. Jesus required certain acts of obedience from him in order to receive healing.

It is a common misconception that it takes much more faith to be healed instantly and supernaturally of a disease than to seek healing with the help of a physician. And many wrongly believe that if a person has to seek a physician for help in dealing with the symptoms of a disease, his or her faith has failed. But really, is it harder or easier to trust God when you see immediate results? I believe it sometimes requires greater faith for us to walk through an illness and seek God's face to find our pathway to healing than it does to receive an instant, miraculous healing from God. We have only to look at the heroes in the Scriptures to know that our faith was meant to take us *through* some difficult situations, not just to keep us *from* them.

HEALING ANOINTING FLOWS THROUGH NATURAL SUBSTANCES

The minute Jesus touched the two blind men in Matthew 20 and the blind man in John 9, His anointing was released into them to effect their healing. They suffered from the same condition—blindness—and in the end, their healings were exactly the same—they could see. But the paths they took to get there were quite different.

When Jesus created the mixture of mud and saliva, it became an anointed salve for the blind man's eyes. Note that the mixture was made of natural things of this earth—mud and saliva. In that sense it is not unlike many medications and treatments we use today; they are natural, made from the earth, and within the realm of man's understanding. However, when Jesus touched that natural mixture of mud and saliva, He anointed it with His healing power. Then He gave the man instructions to go and wash in the Pool of Siloam.

God's pathway to healing will always involve an element of faith to receive His healing power through spiritual or natural means. And it will include instructions that are specifically tailored to the individual. He knows what each person needs and what will most effectively bring about that person's total healing.

Many suggestions in this book are natural remedies that can often provide better results than traditional medicine—and *with fewer or no side effects!* It may surprise you to know that 50 percent of medications approved in recent years are derived from natural products.[1] They are His provision for our healing, as suggested by Scripture:

> The leaves of the tree were for the healing of the nations.
> —REVELATION 22:2

A PROPER PERSPECTIVE

As a Christian physician I cannot view medicine and faith as contradictory issues. Healing received by faith or through medical intervention is not an either-or issue. When a Christian comes to me seeking help with an ailment or disease, I do not consider that his faith has failed. Instead, I consider that through the medical knowledge we gain through diagnosis, we have important tools to help us target our prayers against the specific enemy that has brought disease to the patient's body. Such knowledge helps the patient and me find the pathway to healing that God ordains for him or her. All knowledge comes from God, and He has instructed us to acknowledge Him in all our ways so that He can direct our paths (Prov. 3:6).

The most important key to finding a solution to your illness is to seek God's pathway to healing for *you*—the set of instructions that He has specifically ordained for you to follow that will ultimately set you free from the effects of disease. Chances are it will not be the same pathway as the one God has for your friend, your neighbor, or even another family member. He has a plan specifically suited for you and you alone. You have been fearfully and wonderfully made (Ps. 139)! There is no other creature like you, and your Creator knows exactly what to do to heal your body.

CHAPTER 4

PRAYER—THE BIBLE'S ULTIMATE HEALTH SECRET

The effective, fervent prayer of a righteous man accomplishes much.

—JAMES 5:16

PRAYER IS A potent weapon against disease. Many patients and doctors today are frustrated by their inability to effectively prevent or halt the progression of disease. Even with all of the technological advances in medicine and health care in the last several decades, mankind has not been able to eradicate the presence of illness. Even the common cold is still prevalent, not to mention the major killers stalking us—cardiovascular disease, cancer, and diabetes, just to name a few.

THE EFFECTIVE WEAPON OF PRAYER

In the face of these overwhelming odds what are we to do? As a Christian physician I can tell you that my primary weapon against disease is prayer. When I see patients who are ravaged by the effects of a particular illness—or even worse, their test results and case history are inconclusive so that we are not sure what is causing the symptoms—I do not turn first to further testing or to my prescription pad. I turn to what I consider to be the Bible's greatest health secret: the effective weapon of prayer.

Doctors are only human, and the medical community has limited options. What are you to do when a doctor has done everything he knows to do, tried every treatment available and prescribed every possible medication, but still you do not improve?

Many people who are adrift in the world without God or His Word begin to lose hope and despair that they will ever recover. But as a Christian, you need never lose hope. You should always turn to the almighty God, the One who created your body and who knows how to fix it. He created this world and all the natural remedies available in it, and He sent His Son to purchase your healing with His very blood. This powerful, loving God is on your side! And when you turn to Him, He will always be with you and give you the answer to your deepest needs. The apostle Paul declared this wonderful reality:

> For I am persuaded that neither death nor life, neither angels nor principalities nor powers, neither things present nor things to come, neither height nor depth, nor any other created thing, shall be able to separate us from the love of God, which is in Christ Jesus our Lord.
> —ROMANS 8:38–39

"I DON'T KNOW HOW TO PRAY"

Everyone will face a moment of crisis, a midnight hour, at some point in his or her life. For some the moment comes sooner than for others, but rest assured, your moment will come. What will happen at that time? Will you know what to do? Will you know how to pray?

When many of my patients are faced with serious health crises, they don't know what to do or how to pray effectively. They haven't been prepared for this dark moment. Fortunately God, in His wisdom and providence, has given us in His Word the answers we need for all of life's situations. When my patients ask me to help them pray, I happily show them what the Bible teaches.

In fact, Jesus's disciples asked Him the very question that my patients ask me. They had seen their master's prayer life—the many times that He would retreat to be alone with His Father and pray, sometimes all night—and they saw the power and effectiveness with which He healed the masses. For that reason, they came to Him one day, entreating Him, "Lord, teach us to pray" (Luke 11:1). Jesus provided them with the pattern of prayer that we still use today called the Lord's Prayer.

I believe that Jesus gave this prayer to the disciples—and to us today—not only for us to memorize and recite, but also to teach us the basic principles of prayer. This simple prayer embodies certain fundamentals that we should understand and apply to all our prayers. As we focus briefly on these important aspects of effective prayer, I encourage you to begin to use them in your prayers with renewed faith.

"*Our Father which art in heaven, Hallowed be thy name*" (Matt. 6:9, KJV). We must begin our prayer by acknowledging God as our Father. In His great love, He is our provider, the One who knows us and knows what we need and what is best for us. He is interested in our welfare and is lovingly approachable to His children at any time.

"*Thy kingdom come, Thy will be done in earth, as it is in heaven*" (v. 10,

KJV). As the ultimate "higher power," God's kingdom supersedes—and overrides—all earthly governments. As we learn to recognize that His will is always good, we seek to follow Him always and desire His direction for our lives.

"Give us this day our daily bread" (v. 11, KJV). God is the source for everything we need in our lives on a daily basis. We should ask Him specifically to provide for our needs—including health and healing for every part of our being.

"And forgive us our debts, as we forgive our debtors" (v. 12, KJV). The word *debts* is sometimes translated as "transgressions" or "trespasses." God's perfection can obliterate our imperfections, His wisdom far exceeds ours, and His divine mercy and grace are able to save to the uttermost when we seek forgiveness for our sins. It is important to remember that we are forgiven when we forgive others. (See Matthew 6:14–15.)

"And lead us not into temptation, but deliver us from evil" (v. 13, KJV). There is evil as well as good in the world, and there are things that we may be tempted to do (such as smoking, drinking excessively, or having gluttonous eating habits) that could adversely affect our health and our ability to ward off disease. Only with God's active help that we entreat through prayer can we overcome the many pitfalls, problems, temptations, and opposition that we will inevitably confront.

"For thine is the kingdom, and the power, and the glory, for ever. Amen" (v. 13, KJV). Our success in prayer, in our lives, and in our health will depend on us understanding and remembering who God is, what He asks of us, and how we cultivate relationship with Him.

With this guidance received from Jesus's example, it seems easier to understand how God wants you to pray. But how can you apply this type of prayer to those troubled and confusing times of illness and disease? Below I have listed five specific ways you can pray for your healing when you need it the most.

FIVE WAYS TO PRAY FOR YOUR HEALING

When you or a loved one is faced with a terrible disease, what is the first thing you should do? To whom should you turn? The psalmist declared, "God is our refuge and strength, a very present help in trouble" (Ps. 46:1, KJV). The psalms are filled with prayers and cries from people in desperate trouble who rejoiced when God heard their cries and delivered them. You may turn to those prayers and pray them in your hour of need as well, expecting your loving heavenly Father to answer you as well. But sometimes it is difficult to know exactly how to pray specifically in times of crisis. Here are five effective ways I have found to pray when you are facing a health crisis.

1. Pray for openness to hear God's voice.

After a diagnosis you may be overwhelmed with unsolicited advice from well-meaning friends or loved ones or from someone who has faced a similar illness. You may also face confusing decisions as to which tests or procedures to undergo or which medical options to pursue. Your doctor may be biased toward a certain treatment option and may be pressuring you to make decisions for which you feel unprepared.

The first step to take at such a time is to pray for God's voice to cut through the din of all other voices and clearly make Himself and His will known. His way will provide the greatest peace and can direct you toward the most effective path for your healing.

2. Pray to know how to pray.

Sometimes the confusion can be so great that you may feel at a loss to know how to pray for your healing. The Holy Spirit is your heavenly guide—your instructor in the things of God (John 16:13). He is willing and available to show you how to pray. Begin to spend time waiting on God, and ask the Holy Spirit to give you the words to pray.

3. Pray for correct understanding of Scripture.

When you understand what God's Word has to say about health and healing, and God's role in that healing process, you will become more effective in your prayers. There are three major biblical truths about healing that you need to accept when seeking God for healing.

First, you must first understand that *God wants you to be healed!* Read the following scriptures and allow them to sink deep into your heart, building your faith for healing:

+ "I am the LORD who heals you" (Exod. 15:26).
+ "I will remove sickness from your midst" (Exod. 23:25).
+ "The LORD will take away from you all sickness" (Deut. 7:15).
+ "He sent His word and healed them" (Ps. 107:20).
+ "'I will restore health to you, and I will heal you of your wounds,' says the LORD" (Jer. 30:17).
+ "He…healed all who were sick" (Matt. 8:16).

+ "They will lay hands on the sick, and they will recover" (Mark 16:18).

+ "By His wounds you were healed" (1 Pet. 2:24).

Second, agree to accept the biblical truth that *the price for your healing has already been paid*—by Jesus Christ on the cross! When Jesus came to Earth, mankind faced not one but two tremendous needs: we were hopelessly sinful in heart, and our bodies desperately needed healing. Strange as it may seem, while all Christians believe that Christ died on the cross to redeem mankind from sin, some are not sure about God's provision for healing. They have never understood that on the same day Jesus was crucified, He also took upon Himself our sicknesses, providing redemption for the body of man as well as his soul.

If we believe in salvation—through Christ's sacrifice on the cross to forgive our sins—then, according to the Scriptures, we must believe in physical healing as well. The Bible declares of Christ's death: "He Himself took our infirmities and bore our sicknesses" (Matt. 8:17). The terrible price Christ paid on Calvary bought our physical healing as well as our salvation from sin.

Third, the Bible teaches us to *persevere in prayer*. Too often we expect to receive answers from God instantly, and if they do not appear immediately, we pout and say that God did not hear us. But, as I have mentioned, Jesus taught us to persevere in our prayer efforts. In Luke 18 He told a parable of an unjust judge to illustrate His point. The first verse of that chapter tells us, "And he spake a parable unto them to this end, that men ought always to pray, and not to faint" (kjv). Then He told of a judge who neither feared God nor regarded man. When a widow came to him seeking justice, he ignored her at first, but she kept coming back and crying out to him. Finally the judge said, "Though I fear not God, nor regard man; yet because this widow troubleth me, I will avenge her, lest by her continual coming she weary me" (Luke 18:4–5, kjv).

We must not think we are twisting God's arm to get an answer; He is not an unjust judge. The Scriptures are clear that we often wrestle against unseen enemies that do not give in easily in their desire to defeat us. (See Daniel 10; Ephesians 6.) Jesus's point was this: "And shall not God avenge his own elect, which cry day and night unto him, though he bear long with them? I tell you that he will avenge them speedily" (Luke 18:7–8, kjv). God places a high premium on developing perseverance in His children so that they can defeat the most stubborn enemy.

Have you prayed to be healed and the answer has not come? Pray again, and keep on praying. Don't give up. Be persistent. How often should you pray, and how long should you persevere? The Bible says, "Pray without ceasing" (1 Thess. 5:17). And again, "Praying always with all prayer and supplication in the Spirit, and watching thereunto with all perseverance" (Eph. 6:18, KJV). Be patient. Be faithful. Be determined. Keep praying and believing, and persevere until the answer comes.

4. Specifically target your prayers against your disease.

Become informed about your illness. Learn as many specifics as you can. This is where your doctor can help. Arm yourself against the enemy with as much information as you can gather, and then actively pray, using that information to your advantage. For instance, if your doctor tells you that a specific artery near your heart is becoming blocked and causing cardiovascular difficulties, then pray specifically for that particular artery, that it would become clear, in the name of Jesus! Or if there is a cancerous growth in your body, find out specifically where it is, and then continually lay your hands on that part of your body, commanding the cancer to shrink and disappear.

5. Pray for your own individual pathway to healing.

Perhaps most importantly, pray for God to make clear His pathway to healing—the path that He has designed specifically for you. Use the knowledge from your doctor and from advice given in later chapters of this book to direct you. Bring the options that your doctor presents to you before the throne of grace, and ask the Father which way He would have you to go. Remember, God wants you to be healed! As you acknowledge Him, He will give you His peace and will guide you with His Holy Spirit into the way you should go.

PRAY IN FAITH

I considered writing prayers for each specific condition dealt with in this book, but God stopped me. I believe prayer is the strongest weapon a believer has against the attacks of the enemy, so why would God stop me? I asked Him, curious for the answer. He answered that people must pray in faith and pray with understanding (1 Cor. 14:15). Prayer, to accomplish much, must be effective and fervent (James 5:16). I did not write prayers because if you merely speak my words, they may become empty phrases. Use the principles in this chapter to pray effective and fervent prayers for yourself in truth and understanding.

YOUR DIET AND HOW IT AFFECTS YOUR HEALTH

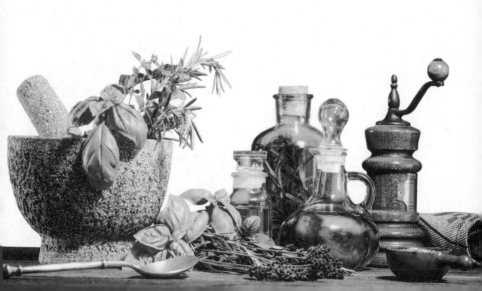

CHAPTER 5

GOD'S NUTRITION

The LORD will take away from you all sickness.

—DEUTERONOMY 7:15

WHEN THE BIBLE speaks to the issue of the healing of our physical bodies, it illustrates clearly a supernatural aspect and a natural aspect of divine health. There are natural, practical things that God wants us to do in order to walk in divine health.

In Exodus 23:25 God said that He would "bless your bread and your water, and I will remove sickness from your midst." This clearly indicates that the practical aspects of people's nutrition contribute prominently in being free of sickness. Let's take a look at nutrition from a biblical perspective.

In the fifteenth chapter of Exodus God entered into a healing covenant with man:

> He said, "If you diligently listen to the voice of the LORD your God, and do what is right in His sight, and give ear to His commandments, and keep all His statutes, I will not afflict you with any of the diseases with which I have afflicted the Egyptians. For I am the LORD who heals you."
> —EXODUS 15:26

Immediately after establishing this covenant of healing with His people, in the sixteenth chapter of Exodus God addressed the issue of nutrition by providing manna to His people. This supernatural, nutritionally sound substance sustained the Israelites for the forty years that they wandered in the wilderness.

When the Israelites reached the Promised Land, they discovered a land rich in nutrition, filled with all the natural provisions of God to enable them to develop the sound, nutritious meal plan that has today become known as the Mediterranean Diet.

The things we eat have always had a direct bearing on the condition of our health. Four of the ten leading causes of death in this country today deal with the issue of what we eat.[1]

GOD'S REASON FOR NUTRITION LAWS

As we just discussed, God made a healing covenant with His people, but then in the next chapter (Exodus 16) He inexplicably began describing in detail what nutritional practices the Israelites were to follow. This shows that for God, and therefore for us, there is a correlation between our health and our nutrition.

It is only recent research that is pointing us to God's reason for and emphasis on nutrition. A singular concept is emerging that is a common thread for all the major diseases facing man today. That single concept is inflammation, and God's dietary guidelines are meant to help us avoid that.

INFLAMMATION AND DIET

Chronic inflammation causes damage to your body over time, but you won't always know about it. You generally won't be able to feel its effects, but it can be part of the cause of many diseases and conditions common in America today, including diabetes, depression, heart disease, and others.[2]

The typical American diet only plays into this; it actually leads directly to chronic inflammation. Trans fats, sugar, artificial sweeteners, and many more common products in the diet of most Americans can increase the level of inflammation in your body. This means fried and fast foods, baked goods, and even white bread can lead to inflammation. Advanced glycation end products (AGEs), another product commonly consumed through dairy, sugar, and meats cooked at very high temperatures, are linked to inflammation and can cause diseases such as heart disease and diabetic complications. Omega-6s, found commonly in foods containing corn oil or hydrogenated oils, can produce hormones that cause inflammation.[3]

This can sound daunting. Each of these products can be difficult to avoid today, but remember God has given us guidelines on healthy foods through His Word. We will discuss more specific diet plans later in the book, but here are some basic guidelines for foods that cause inflammation and foods that fight inflammation.

INFLAMMATORY EFFECT OF FOODS

Decrease Inflammation	Increase Inflammation
Corn oil	Vegetables
Peanut oil	Canola oil
Processed lunch meats	Olive oil
Steak/full fat animal meats	Fish
Hamburger	Cereals
White rice	Dark bread
Pastries	Oatmeal
Fries	Walnuts
Pasta	Bran
Low-grain (white) bread	Almonds
	Flaxseed
	Chia seed
	Brown rice
	Sweet potatoes
	Beans
	Legumes

CHAPTER 6

THE FALLACY OF FAD DIETS

Bless the LORD, O my soul, and forget not all His benefits...who satisfies your mouth with good things, so that your youth is renewed like the eagle's.

—PSALM 103:2, 5

IT'S NO SECRET that the general American public is increasingly more overweight. In fact, there seems to be a direct correlation in the last decade or so between the size of our cars (sport utility vehicles), the size of our meals ("Could you super-size that?"), and the size of our waistlines! In 1980, 46 percent of adults in the United States age twenty or older were overweight or obese; by 1999 the number had increased to 65 percent. In 2013, 70 percent of adult Americans were either overweight or obese.[1]

We all know that it's not good to be overweight. But it's not just a matter of how we look. Did you know that being just ten to twenty pounds overweight increases your risk of premature death?[2] Those excess pounds increase your risk of heart disease, diabetes, cancer, asthma, and other illnesses. In fact, every two-pound increase in weight increases the risk of arthritis by at least 9 percent, and a woman who gains just a pound a year after age twenty can nearly double her chance of postmenopausal breast cancer.[3] I have found a weight gain of *just eleven pounds* will *double* the risk of acquiring type 2 diabetes!

ARE YOU OVERWEIGHT AND AT RISK FOR DISEASE?

A person's body mass index (BMI) and waist circumference are two useful indicators for determining whether he or she is at increased risk for health problems associated with being overweight or obese. Generally the higher your BMI (your height to weight ratio), the higher your health risk, and the risk increases if your waist size is greater than thirty-five inches for women or forty inches for men.[4]

Calculate your own risk

To find out if you are overweight and to determine your health risk, first find your BMI. The CDC has a BMI calculator online, or you can simply search the Internet for "BMI Calculator."[5]

Check your BMI in the chart below to measure your health risk relative to normal weight:[6]

BMI		Waist Less Than or Equal to 35" (Women) or 40" (Men)	Waist Greater than 35" (Women) or 40" (Men)
18.5 or less	Underweight	Low risk	Low risk
18.6–24.9	Normal	Low risk	Low risk
25.0–29.9	Overweight	Increased risk	High risk
30.0–34.9	Obese	High risk	Very high risk
35.0–39.9	Obese	Very high risk	Very high risk
40.0 or greater	Extremely obese	Extremely high risk	Extremely high risk

If you think you need to start dieting, you are not alone. The public's awareness of this widening problem (no pun intended!) has increased dramatically in the last several years, as evidenced by the number of fad diets being promoted almost every time you turn on the television set. People want to lose the weight! According to the Boston Medical Center, there are 45 million Americans who diet each year.[7] But just who has the right plan? Is the new concept of low-carb, high-fat diets really a dream come true? Or is a low-fat diet the answer?

Finding the true solution that will work for you requires cutting through the confusion that is presently in the public forum on this issue and taking a look at the facts. Let's consider some of the most popular diets that are on the market today.

"FAD" DIETS

The age-old theme of "eat less and exercise more" hasn't been popular enough to launch any diet book onto the best-seller list. What does sell, however, is any book that promises some new miracle or breakthrough method for easy weight loss. While there may be one or two good points about each of the new popular fad diets on the market today, by and large, they don't produce long-term results. They may even prove to be risky to your health rather than beneficial.

Most of these diets are based on the principle of monitoring two metabolic hormones, insulin and glucagon, and the regulation of glucose, the blood sugar that all carbohydrates will eventually become. Because the brain needs glucose to survive, there must be a certain amount of it present at all times. However, because high blood glucose levels (hyperglycemia) are damaging to the body, insulin, which decreases blood glucose, and glucagon, which increases it, regulate the levels.

After you eat a meal, glucose floods the bloodstream and the pancreas secretes insulin, which brings the blood glucose levels back down to normal. Glucagon has the opposite effect: if blood glucose levels get too low, it will signal the release of glucose from other storage sites (primarily the liver) to keep the brain in full supply. This happens frequently at night when you are sleeping. Because you go for several hours without eating, the supply of glucose for the brain must come from somewhere within the body, which the glucagon works to supply.

Another concept important for understanding the major diet books is the glycemic index. This index measures how quickly certain foods (carbohydrates) are digested and become present in the bloodstream as glucose. Foods such as white bread, pure sugar, pasta, and potatoes are more quickly digested (higher glycemic index) than foods such as beans or wheat bread. The proposed problem with foods with a higher glycemic index is that they can cause a rapid rise in glucose and a greater insulin response in the body. However, the glycemic index only accounts for foods eaten isolated from each other, not those eaten together in a meal.

Armed with these facts, you will be able to understand the functioning principles of the following dietary regimens.

Dr. Atkins's New Diet Revolution

This popular yet controversial diet is based on the premise that people who are overweight are actually experiencing an overreaction of insulin to the carbohydrates that they eat. In people who have a large insulin response, blood glucose falls rapidly, causing hunger and resulting in overeating. To break this cycle Atkins proposes a high-fat, low-carbohydrate diet, claiming that by increasing the fat in the diet, people will eat less because of the feeling of fullness that the fat can promote. However, carbohydrates are drastically restricted in the hope that insulin levels will stabilize and hunger will be suppressed. The additional benefit is that since the brain needs glucose to survive, if it does not get what it needs from carbohydrates in the diet, the body will begin to break down fat cells as an alternate energy source.

Fallacy: There is no scientific proof that high insulin levels cause weight gain. There is, however, scientific proof that a diet high in saturated fats will increase the risk of heart disease and some forms of cancer. As the body burns its own fat reservoirs to make up for what is lacking in the diet, high levels of needed electrolytes such as calcium, potassium, and sodium are lost in the urine. Because these are not being replaced in the diet, many potential problems are the result, including cardiac arrhythmia, osteoporosis, nausea, light-headedness, and fatigue.

Many people claim to have lost weight on Dr. Atkins's diet plan (as well as similar diet plans, such as the ketogenic diet), and that may be true, but it is a weight loss primarily due to a rapid loss of body fluids (needed to excrete the waste created from burning the body's own fat resources). This one premise can cause a host of other health concerns, including kidney problems.

The Ornish diet

Dr. Dean Ornish designed his diet plan to help patients reduce their risk of heart disease through full-sweeping lifestyle changes. His diet is a low-fat one, with reduced protein but increased consumption of whole foods, fruits, vegetables, grains, beans, and soy products. The Ornish diet has the most scientific support for its success in promoting weight loss. The main problem with it is gaining compliance. Its extreme limitations on fat often prove too difficult for any but the most dedicated and disciplined dieter to follow.

The Zone diet

The Zone diet is better known as the 30/30/40 diet, in which 30 percent of daily calories come from fat, 30 percent from protein and 40 percent from carbohydrates. These percentages were calculated to be the "optimal" ratio to control something called *eicosanoids*, hormonelike compounds in the body thought to be involved in inflammation and certain diseases. It remains an open question as to whether this diet has any effect on eicosanoids or any disease process, but what is certain is that it restricts many foods in the fruits and vegetables category, which are known for their beneficial effects on health.

Sugar busters

The sugar buster diet proclaims, predictably, that all sugar is toxic to the human body. Therefore, foods that are high on the glycemic index are eliminated, and other foods low on the scale, such as whole grains, vegetables, fruits, lean meat, and fiber, are consumed instead. The problem with this diet is that while it is reducing a person's sugar intake, other nutritious foods are eliminated, such as carrots, beets, and potatoes. If you decide to follow this diet, chances are that you will lose weight, but you will open yourself up to greater health risks due to lacking nutrients. As with the Ornish diet, many people who begin the sugar busters diet start strong, but they cannot maintain it for any length of time due to its rigidity.

TRUTH ABOUT FAD DIETS

Most of the new fad diets that are on the market today are actually harmful to a person's health. They tend to run to one extreme or the other, containing excessive amounts of cholesterol, saturated fat, or animal protein. They also tend to be lacking in many key nutrients necessary to counter disease. Other potential dangerous effects that have been noted include:

+ Mild dehydration
+ Headaches
+ Nausea
+ Sleep problems
+ Fatigue
+ Increased risk of osteoporosis
+ Inability to maintain weight loss
+ High blood pressure

FREEDOM FROM FAD DIETS

So what is a person to do? I have good news: through the combination of eating the right foods, burning calories through physical exercise, and supplementing the diet with the proper nutrients, it is possible to lose weight and keep it off! And not only can you do it without any detrimental effects to your body, but also your health will actually improve as a result of the changes that you make.

Foods that increase metabolism

As scientists continue to study the chemistry of the human body, five common groups of foods have been proven to increase metabolism and block the fatty acid uptake in the body's cells, thus causing a person to lose weight.

1. *Oatmeal.* The fiber found in common oatmeal has an incredible impact on the insulin levels in the bloodstream. When you eat sugary foods, the insulin converts those carbohydrates into fat storage and slows down your metabolism. But the fiber present in oatmeal blunts that insulin response. Anyone who is struggling to lose weight should fix themselves a bowl of oatmeal, or another type of oat bran cereal that is high in fiber, for breakfast. Fiber supplements such as apple pulp concentrate, citrus pectin, and glucomannan, from the konjac plant, can also have the same effect.

2. *Salsa.* Spicy foods such as salsa, jalapeño peppers, and cayenne peppers have been shown to increase the body's metabolism and burn more calories, even when the body is at rest. The chemical capsaicin, which actually causes the spiciness, is the key. One study showed that a single spicy meal increased people's metabolism by 25 percent, and the effect lasted for three hours.[8] I mention salsa in particular because the tomatoes contain lycopene, another helpful component in the prevention of breast cancer and prostate cancer.[9]

3. *Green tea.* Certain chemicals within the green teas commonly found in Asian countries have been shown to increase the body's metabolic rate and increase the breakdown and elimination of fat. The polyphenols present in the tea have a *thermogenic effect* on the body; that is, they cause the body to begin to burn its fat reservoirs. The amount of caffeine that is present in green tea doesn't cause the jitters, unlike the amount found in coffee, but it does increase metabolism and allows the body to burn more calories while resting.

4. *Protein.* Diets that restrict protein intake are missing one important fact: protein requires more calories to digest in the body than do carbohydrates or fats. To a certain extent, shifting to a higher protein diet will burn more calories and cause you to lose more weight. It is important not to go to an

extreme with this, however, because too much protein can be harmful to the kidneys. It is also better to obtain protein in your diet from low-fat sources such as poultry and fish rather than from red meats.

5. *Fish.* The omega-3 fatty acids present in fish such as salmon, trout, mackerel, cod, and sardines have consistently been shown to increase body metabolism.

Increased body metabolism is important because it increases the rate at which the body can burn fat while at rest. In other words, you can be "working off" those calories just by sitting in your chair! In fact, approximately 70 percent of the total calories that you burn are burned while at rest, just to keep the heart beating, your intestines working, your food being digested in your system, and other "automatic" processes, according to the Mayo Clinic.[10] However, if you hope to lose weight and maintain good health, burning metabolic calories alone is not enough. Physical activity should be an important factor in any weight-loss plan.

Burning calories through exercise

Different types of physical exercise will burn more or fewer calories depending on the effort that is exerted. When I get out and run a seven-minute mile, I burn about 984 calories per hour. Walking at a moderate pace will burn about 246 calories per hour.

My wife, Linda, burns a lot of calories just working around the house. When she has to climb up and down the ladder to install the rain gutters around the house, she is burning 422 calories an hour. When she washes my car, if she does it vigorously enough, she burns 316 calories an hour. And hanging the storm windows causes her to burn 352 calories an hour! Now, of course I don't make my wife do those things, but my point is this: Make exercise a part of your life. Begin to take the stairs rather than the elevator. Park a little farther away from your destination and give yourself the opportunity for a brisk walk. And find a physical activity that suits you that you can stick to regularly.

Did you know that even working at the office can burn calories? Just by sitting at your desk doing paperwork, you burn 127 calories an hour. Taking a nap (sleeping) burns 63 calories an hour. But by far the most strenuous exercise, for those of you who are ready to snap yourself into shape, is cross-country skiing, uphill, which burns 1,160 calories per hour!

Physical activities that will help you control your weight will be the ones that you enjoy and will turn to on a consistent basis.

Natural supplements that promote weight loss

Many people who need to lose weight are intimidated by having to make sudden lifestyle changes such as changing their diets or starting up an intensive exercise program. Because of this, I encourage many of my patients to start simply, to do something they know they can do, such as taking supplements indigenous to the natural plant kingdom that will have a weight-loss effect.

5-HTP (Griffonia)

5-HTP is a naturally occurring chemical found in *Griffonia*, a plant that is native to India. This chemical works differently from other weight-loss products in that it is converted in the human body into the neurotransmitter serotonin. Serotonin has been found to be helpful for people facing memory problems, depression, and anxiety.[11] Lower doses of it will directly work on the hypothalamus gland within the brain, the gland that is responsible for the appetite.

Have you ever noticed that when you receive bad news, your appetite is suddenly gone? Your sudden change in mood has affected the serotonin levels in your brain, which in turn has affected your appetite center. So the benefit of 5-HTP is that it can control the food cravings that many overweight people experience without side effects.

The urge to eat is built within human beings for the purpose of survival. Though it was created by God for a good purpose, God's good plans are often twisted and distorted in our fallen world. What was once a healthy appetite gets out of control, and the deep, almost visceral cravings can get out of hand. If you feel that your food cravings are biological, you are right! But thank God that He has provided a way out of every temptation, and in this case it is through the 5-HTP He has provided in His plant kingdom. A dose of 100 milligrams is a sufficient dose for the purpose of weight loss.

Garcinia (hydroxycitric acid)

A second supplement from the plant kingdom comes from a gourd called a *garcinia*, which looks like a cross between an acorn squash and an orange. It contains the chemical *hydroxycitric acid*, which blocks the conversion of carbohydrates into fat storage. So if you eat too many carbohydrates and they are not burned off as energy, this supplement allows the extra carbohydrates to not be stored as fat as they usually would be.

Instead it turns those carbohydrates into glycogen, a harmless chemical that does not accumulate as fat. You should take a dose of 900 milligrams per day to help you lose weight.

Platycodon

One prescription that is often given by doctors to patients who need to lose weight is Xenical, a drug that decreases fat absorption in the body, but it is often accompanied by side effects such as diarrhea and other problems in the gastrointestinal tract. However, for centuries the plant *platycodon* has existed in China, which is now proving to have the same positive results in fat absorption and weight loss as Xenical, but with none of the negative side effects. Platycodon works by inhibiting the enzyme lipase, which causes the fat to be absorbed. A dose of 100 milligrams of the platycodon root is sufficient for weight loss.

WEIGHT LOSS IS POSSIBLE!

In conclusion it is a myth that it is impossible to succeed at weight loss! According to a paper published in the *American Journal of Clinical Nutrition* in 2005 that tracked the success of weight loss over time, there are individuals who have successfully lost at least 10 percent of their body weight and kept it off, with the average individual losing approximately 70 pounds and keeping it off for five years![12] Their pathway to successful weight loss was through changes in their diets and exercise patterns.

You can succeed despite your genetic profile! Although 70 percent of the people involved in a 1997 study had at least one parent who was significantly overweight, some still saw success in losing and maintaining weight loss.[13]

You can succeed despite your cravings! The people in these studies didn't give up sweets altogether—they just drastically limited their intake. One person ate the icing off of a cupcake and threw the rest of it away. Another person divided ice cream into tiny cubes and ate just one cube a day.

You can succeed without taking harmful "diet drugs" such as ephedra or fen-phen! These people modified their lifestyles rather than sending their bodies on a roller-coaster ride of highs and lows that many diet drugs cause.

You can succeed by finding God's pathway to healing (and weight loss) designed *just for you!*

ESSENTIAL NUTRIENTS TO ACHIEVE YOUR OPTIMAL WEIGHT		
Natural Substance	**Effect**	**Daily Dosage**
Garcinia	Plant extract that helps suppress appetite and may help block the synthesis of fat in the body	900 mg
Glucomannan	Soluble fiber that slows the absorption of sugars from the intestinal tract, improves blood lipid levels, and helps control appetite	1,500 mg
Inulin	Plant extract with fiber-like qualities that enhances the growth of beneficial intestinal flora	800 mg
Green tea leaf	Herb with important antioxidant activity and phytochemicals that have been shown to increase the burning of fat for energy	200 mg
5-HTP	Amino acid derivative naturally found in the body that helps elevate mood and suppress the appetite	100 mg
Platycodon root	Herb traditionally used in China and other Asian countries to prevent obesity	100 mg
Cayenne pepper	Herb that may increase amount of calories burned and help control appetite	10 mg

CHAPTER 7

HEALTHY EATING WITH
THE MEDITERRANEAN DIET

A GREAT INTEREST HAS arisen in medical and health circles today about the foods that have been eaten for centuries in the lands of the Bible. The diet of Middle Eastern people is of particular interest.

One name given to this group of foods that prevent disease and help to cure diseases is the "Mediterranean Diet." This diet is very similar to the one described in Genesis.

עַל־פְּנֵי כָל־הָאָרֶץ וְאֶת־כָּל־הָעֵץ אֲשֶׁר־בּוֹ פְרִי־עֵץ זֹרֵעַ זֶרַע לָכֶם וַיֹּאמֶר אֱלֹהִים הִנֵּה נָתַתִּי לָכֶם אֶת־כָּל־עֵשֶׂב זֹרֵעַ זֶרַע אֲשֶׁר. And God said, Behold, I have given you every herb bearing seed, which is upon the face of all the earth, and every tree, in the which is the fruit of a tree yielding seed; to you it shall be for meat.

—GENESIS 1:29, KJV

אֲשֶׁר הוּא־חַי לָכֶם יִהְיֶה לְאָכְלָה כְּיֶרֶק עֵשֶׂב נָתַתִּי לָכֶם אֶת־כֹּל... כָּל־רֶמֶשׂ. Every moving thing that liveth shall be meat for you; even as the green herb have I given you all things.

—GENESIS 9:3, KJV

We will identify some of the specific foods mentioned in the Bible cure throughout the Old and New Covenants, and then observe the foods that are eaten today in those same regions around the Mediterranean Sea. I will list the specific foods mentioned in the Bible cure and then describe more generally the food groups you should eat in order to enjoy the health benefits that are rooted in the Bible cure's Mediterranean Diet.

SPECIFIC FOODS MENTIONED IN THE BIBLE CURE

The Bible cure gives us specific commands about two things: First, we are to avoid certain fats: "It shall be a perpetual statute for your generations...that ye eat neither fat nor blood" (Lev. 3:17, KJV). Second, we are to avoid obesity: "And take heed to yourselves, lest at any time your hearts be overcharged with surfeiting, and drunkenness, and cares of

45

this life, and so that day come upon you unawares. For as a snare shall it come on all them that dwell on the face of the whole earth" (Luke 21:34–35, KJV).

In addition to the foods we are to avoid eating, the Bible cure mentions the following specific foods that are found throughout the Mediterranean Diet and should be the source of food for us today.

+ Clean, lean meat from animals with divided hooves; animals that are cud-chewing (Lev. 11:2–3)
+ Fish with fins *and* scales (Lev. 11:9; Deut. 14:9)
+ Cucumbers, melons, leeks, onions, and garlic (Num. 11:5)
+ Grapes (Deut. 8:7–9; John 15)
+ Wheat, barley, vines (grapes), figs, pomegranates, olive oil, and honey (Deut. 8:8)
+ Raisins and apples (Song of Songs 2:5)
+ Bread (Exod. 12:8, 15; Ezek. 4:9)
+ Beans (Ezek. 4:9)
+ Honey, pistachio nuts, and almonds (Gen. 43:11)
+ Yogurt and the milk of cows, sheep, and goats (Isa. 7:15, 22; Prov. 27:27)

FOODS IN OLD TESTAMENT TIMES

Like many Arabs today, the Hebrews ate meat only on festive occasions. To vary the monotonous daily diet of parched or cooked wheat and barley, the Hebrew housewife would grind the grain into coarse flour, mix it with olive oil, and bake it into flat cakes of bread. She garnished the cakes with lentils, broad beans, and other vegetables. Cucumbers, onions, leeks, and garlic perked up bland dishes. Fresh and dried fruit and wild honey sweetened the meals. In a water-short land the Hebrews heartily quaffed wine and prized the milk of goats and sheep.

Solomon and his sumptuous court demanded richer fare for their golden table: "Solomon's daily provisions were thirty cors of the finest flour and sixty cors of meal, ten head of stall-fed cattle, twenty of pasture-fed cattle and a hundred sheep and goats, as well as deer, gazelles, roebucks and choice fowl" (1 Kings 4:22–23, NIV).

We can even get a glimpse into the everyday life of Mary, Joseph, and Jesus, and we find that their dinner table held many of the same foods as those provided by Solomon to his people:

In her daily rounds she [the Jewish maiden Mary] would have fetched water, tended the fire, and ground grain. The family dined on a porridge of wheat or barley groats, supplemented by beans, lentils, cucumbers, and other vegetables—with onions, leeks, garlic, and olive oil for seasoning. For dessert came dates, figs, and pomegranates. Watered wine was the universal drink. Only on feast days did humble Galileans eat meat.[1]

THE MEDITERRANEAN DIET

The Bible cure identifies some of the basic foods found in the Mediterranean Diet, which offers a healthy basis for eating that is rooted in the truths of the ancient Hebrew texts. Let's examine some of the specific foods eaten by those in the ancient world to see how they help us to prevent and cure disease.

There has been a great interest developing in what is known as the Mediterranean Diet. This diet is very similar to one outlined in Genesis 1:29 and Genesis 9:3. It seems that the diet followed by people living along the Mediterranean Sea results in some of the lowest rates of colon cancer, breast cancer, and coronary heart disease in the world.[2] Why would this be?

It is no accident that Israel is one of these Mediterranean countries. I believe that most of this diet can be traced back to the Bible cure guidelines given to God's chosen people—the Israelites.

Mediterranean countries have developed their own dishes, but these dishes share several characteristics. As you take a look at the ingredients used in these menus, you will observe that the following foods are consumed frequently:

1. *Olive oil.* Olive oil replaces most fats, oils, butter, and margarine; it is used in salads as well as for cooking. Olive oil raises levels of the good cholesterol (HDL) and may strengthen immune system function. Extra-virgin olive oil is preferred.

2. *Vegetables and fruits.* Try to eat between seven and ten serving of fruits and veggies each day. Dark green vegetables are prominent, especially in salads. To obtain the same benefits in our diet, we should eat at least one of the following vegetables daily: cabbage, broccoli, cauliflower, turnip greens, or mustard greens. The Mediterranean Diet includes many fruits, preferably raw. Eat two to three servings daily. Eat one of the

following vegetables or fruits daily: carrots, spinach, sweet potatoes, cantaloupe, peaches, or apricots.

3. *Fish.* The healthiest fish are cold-water varieties such as cod, salmon, and tuna; trout is also good. These fish are high in omega-3 fatty acids. Eat fish twice a week.

4. *Poultry.* Poultry can be eaten two to three times weekly; white breast meat from which the skin has been removed is the best.

5. *Grains.* The Mediterranean Diet includes many sources of grains. To obtain the same healthy grains, eat cereals containing wheat bran (one-half cup, four to five times weekly); alternate with a cereal such as Bran Buds (one-half cup) or one that contains oat bran (one-third cup).

6. *Breads.* Bread is consumed daily in small amounts and is prepared as dark, chewy, crusty loaves. The typical American sliced white bread and wheat breads are not used in the Mediterranean countries.

7. *Beans.* The Mediterranean Diet includes many kinds of beans, including pintos, great northern, navy, and kidney beans. Bean and lentil soups are very popular (prepared with a small amount of olive oil). We should have at least one-half cup of beans, three to four times weekly.

8. *Nuts.* Almonds (ten per day) or walnuts (ten per day) rank at the top of the list of acceptable nuts in the Mediterranean Diet.

9. *Cheese and yogurt.* Recent studies indicate that cheese may not contribute as much to clogged arteries as was previously believed. In fact, an article published in *Current Nutrition Reports* shows that the consumption of dairy products, including cheese and yogurt, actually reduces the risk of heart disease.[3] In the Mediterranean Diet cheese may be grated on soups, or a small wedge may be combined with a piece of fruit for dessert; use the reduced-fat varieties (the fat-free often taste like rubber). The best yogurt is fat-free, but not frozen.

10. *Pasta, rice, couscous, bulgur, potatoes.* Pasta is usually a side dish containing no more than 1 cup of pasta. It is often served with fresh vegetables and herbs sautéed in olive oil; occasionally it is served with small quantities of lean beef. Dark rice is preferred. Couscous and bulgur are other forms of wheat.

In addition to these healthy foods that are included in the Mediterranean Diet on a daily basis, there are some foods that should be included in your diet, but only a few times weekly or less. These include:

1. *Eggs.* Eggs should be eaten in small amounts (two to three per week).

2. *Red meat.* Red meat should only be included in your diet on an average of three times a month. Use only lean cuts with the fat trimmed; it can also be used in small amounts as an additive to spice up soup or pasta. The severe restriction of red meat in the Mediterranean Diet is a radical departure from the American diet, but it is a major contributor to the low rates of cancer and heart disease found in these countries.

EATING THE MEDITERRANEAN WAY

A typical Mediterranean breakfast would consist of dark bread or cereal (such as those mentioned), a piece of fresh fruit, and perhaps a small amount of yogurt or a slice of cheese. Lunch or dinner would very likely include:

1. *Salads.* The salad is eaten with each meal; it is made of fresh greens (and other vegetables) with added olive oil, vinegar, and/ or lemon juice.

2. *Soups.* Soups are often made with chopped celery, garlic, carrots, onions, and other vegetables and cooked in a chicken stock or other liquid. They are seasoned with added herbs; a small amount of grated cheese (use low-fat) is sprinkled for garnish on top.

3. *Pasta.* A side of fresh pasta is often mixed with fresh vegetables and herbs that have been sautéed in olive oil. Occasionally a bit of beef or chicken is added.

4. *Rice.* Rice is a prominent addition in this diet. Many different rices are used, including the dark, brown, and wild rices. These are prepared in many creative ways, including rice pilafs, risottos, and thick soups and stews.

5. *Staple items.* Many fruits and vegetables are staples in the Mediterranean Diet. Tomatoes, onions, and peppers are used

often. Olive oil is used often in cooking and salads instead of
heavy oils.

THE MEDITERRANEAN FOOD PYRAMID

The food pyramid summarizes the eating habits of people who eat the
Mediterranean way. In the pages following the pyramid, notice the balance between the amounts of each category of food in this diet.

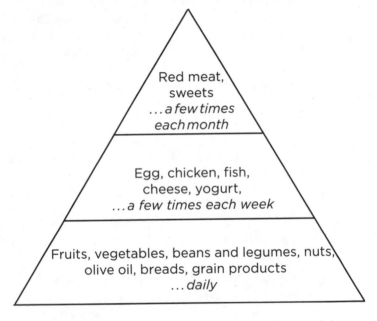

Red meat,
sweets
*...a few times
each month*

Egg, chicken, fish,
cheese, yogurt,
...a few times each week

Fruits, vegetables, beans and legumes, nuts,
olive oil, breads, grain products
...daily

The Mediterranean Diet Food Pyramid

A "NEW WINE" FOR YOUR HEALTH

There have been more than fifty research articles from universities indicating the health benefits of wine (particularly red wine). Since the Bible
talks so much about wine, Linda and I researched the subject and discovered that red wine contains a useful substance (resveratrol). Researchers
at the University of Illinois have found that resveratrol inhibits cancer
by helping to prevent DNA damage to cells, keeping cells from trans-
forming into cancer and thus preventing the growth and spread of
cancer.[4] In recent Cornell University studies resveratrol has been shown
to lower cholesterol.

Other substances in red wine known as biologically active flavonoids are potent antioxidants. Antioxidants neutralize free radicals, which may be the root cause of cancer, heart disease, cataracts, rheumatoid arthritis, and the aging process itself. Flavonoids can also protect us from strokes and heart attacks by reducing platelet aggregation, which allows the blood to flow more smoothly through the blood vessels.

God, in His infinite wisdom, has now shown us how to get the benefits of wine without the alcohol; Linda and I use a nonalcoholic red wine made by Ariel (a type of wine known as a Cabernet Sauvignon). Go to www.arielvineyards.com for information. You should drink six to twelve ounces daily to gain the benefits mentioned above. The thought of drinking "wine" is foreign to many, but without the alcohol we can obtain all the benefits God intended without the detriments.

Pray about this; God may use this as a part of your pathway to healing and health.

WHAT SHOULD I BE EATING?

We have already looked at some of the foods that are healthy for us. Let's look again, this time considering the essential nutrient compounds for a healthy diet and the foods that provide each nutrient to our body.

Protein

While protein is essential to our health, we should limit our protein intake to 10 to 15 percent of our total calories. Excessive amounts of protein can lead to kidney problems, high cholesterol levels, and heart disease, as well as other health-related problems.

Limit red meats to three servings monthly. Emphasize fish (especially trout, salmon, cod, and tuna) and chicken (preferably white meat without skin).

Carbohydrates

God set the pattern for our nutritional intake in the Book of Genesis:

> Then God said, "See, I have given you every plant yielding seed which is on the face of all the earth and every tree which has fruit yielding seed. It shall be food for you."
>
> —GENESIS 1:29

> Every moving thing that lives will be food for you. I give you everything, just as I gave you the green plant.
>
> —GENESIS 9:3

The verse from the first chapter of Genesis above deals with the natural foods God gave us to meet our nutritive need for carbohydrates. Grains, seeds, fruits, and vegetables are the sources we have available to us for carbohydrates.

Complex carbohydrates are vitally important to our healthy bodies. There are some people groups in the world today (particularly in Asian countries) where hardening of the arteries and cancer are almost nonexistent—due to a diet consisting primarily of complex carbohydrates.

Most of your food should be from the following list of complex carbohydrates:

+ *Green/yellow vegetables*—three or more servings daily
+ *Grains, including cereal, rice, whole-grain breads*—two servings daily
+ *Fruits*—three or more daily
+ *Beans and peas*—three servings weekly

Certain carbohydrate-rich vegetables and fruits show cancer-protective effects. These include:

+ *Those high in vitamin A*
  These fruits and vegetables are often orange or yellow in color. They include apricots, carrots, cantaloupe, pumpkin, peaches, and sweet potatoes. Other very good complex-carbohydrate sources are watermelon, broccoli, collard greens, romaine lettuce, and tomatoes.

+ *Those high in vitamin C*
  Vitamin C–rich food sources include cantaloupe, broccoli, collard greens, oranges, cabbage, tomatoes, strawberries, cauliflower, and spinach.

+ *Cruciferous vegetables*
  Eat at least some of these vegetables several times a week. They include broccoli, cabbage, brussels sprouts, cauliflower, and kale.

Carbohydrates are mentioned frequently in the Bible. One of the best examples of a high complex-carbohydrate diet in the Bible cure can be seen in the example of Daniel. When Daniel and his friends refused to eat the rich, fat-laden, unhealthy foods from the king's table, Daniel appealed to the king's steward for a different menu:

> Then said Daniel to the steward... "Please test your servants for ten days, and let them give us vegetables to eat and water to drink. Then let our countenances be looked upon before you, and the countenance of the youths who eat of the portion of the king's food. And as you see, deal with your servants." So he consented to them in this matter and tested them for ten days. At the end of ten days their countenances appeared fairer and fatter than all the youths who ate the portion of the king's food. Thus the guard continued to take away the portion of their food and the wine that they were to drink, and gave them vegetables.
>
> —DANIEL 1:11–16

What a great example Daniel and his friends are of the healthy benefits of a carbohydrate-rich diet.

Fiber

Fiber, an essential portion of your daily diet, comes from many sources, including fruits and vegetables, as well as many grains. Consider some of the following choices for fiber:

+ *Wheat fiber* from bran-type cereals. Wheat fiber has been proven to be successful in preventing certain types of cancer. Try to get one-half cup of bran cereal daily.

+ *Oat fiber (oat bran)* may lower blood-fat levels (cholesterol). Consider including one-third cup of an oat bran cereal daily. (It may be mixed with wheat bran.)

+ *Beans and peas* should be eaten regularly (preferably three times weekly). Include great northern, pinto, limas, and lentils, all of which seem to lower cholesterol (blood fats).

Fats

God's harshest words about nutrition concern fats:

> As a continual statute for your generations in all your settlements, you shall not eat any fat or any blood.
>
> —LEVITICUS 3:17

About one-third of the American diet is fat.[5] We rank among the highest percentage group of people in the world for heart disease and hardening of the arteries. You will need to give close consideration to your fat intake. You can successfully lower your fat consumption and pave the pathway to better health by following these simple guidelines:

+ *Eat lean red meat sparingly.* Emphasize fish and chicken in your diet.

+ *Limit cheese.* Cheese is sometimes more than 50 percent fat; eat skim-milk, low-fat, or nonfat cheeses.

+ *Oils.* Read labels for "palm kernel oil" and avoid these products. Watch out for coffee creamers, artificial dairy toppings, and hydrogenated or partially hydrogenated oils.

Certain types of fat can be good to include in your diet. Substitute these good fats for those that are unhealthy for you to eat. They include:

+ *Canola oil.* This oil may actually lower blood fat levels; use it for cooking, in recipes, and for salad dressings.

+ *Olive oil.* Olive oil is good for you—it may lower blood fats. Some studies suggest that it may also lower blood pressure. Use it on salads, for cooking, as a substitute in many recipes, and in place of margarine.

+ *Certain oily fish.* Fish such as tuna, salmon, and cod may lower the tendency to develop blood clots and heart disease.

Sugar

Be careful with simple sugars; limit them in your diet—they are too high in calories. Sugar-laden desserts are often high in saturated fat. At the present time, sugar substitutes seem to be safe. Aspartame is actually a combination of natural amino acids that occurs in peaches, green beans, milk, and in many common substances. Some people, however, tolerate aspartame poorly and should avoid it, as it can occasionally cause headaches, allergies, and other reactions. Although saccharin seems to be safe, aspartame (small amounts) and stevia are the preferred choices.

Salt

Salt, or sodium chloride, is necessary to our body, but it can be extremely harmful if overused. Do not add salt when you are cooking, and do not add it at the table on prepared food. If you must "spice up" the taste of your food, consider a salt substitute or a "lite" salt. Be creative with some of the herb-combination substitutes available today. Don't use salt tablets—they have no nutritive value to a healthy diet.

Coffee

The caffeine in coffee (in excessive amounts) can increase cholesterol levels, cause heart irregularities, and may contribute to discomfort from fibrocystic disease in women. Limit your coffee intake to two cups of regular coffee daily; the rest should be decaffeinated.

How to Shop for Food

When God entered a healing covenant with man, He immediately shifted the focus to what His people should eat, giving specific instructions as to how they should gather and prepare their food. (See Exodus 15:26.) In Exodus 23:25 God promised to place a blessing on the bread and water (the daily food) of His people. With His blessing, God indicated that He would "remove sickness from your midst."

The Surgeon General of the United States once reaffirmed God's nutritional laws by stating: "Your choice of diet can influence your long-term health prospects more than any other action you might take." [6]

The following section will help you prepare to examine your diet and to determine to choose the foods for you and your family that will bring you the ultimate opportunity for good health. Choose wisely—your health, and that of your family, will be affected by your choices.

Buying fresh produce

+ Add more produce to your diet. There are many varieties from which to choose.

+ Remember that romaine lettuce is the best choice in the lettuce family.

+ Choose produce known to be good sources of vitamin C: peppers, tomatoes, broccoli, cabbage, potatoes, greens (collard, mustard, turnip), cantaloupe, honeydew, kiwi, and strawberries.

+ Eat the skins of fruits and vegetables.

+ Select produce high in vitamin A: deep-colored green, yellow, and orange vegetables; include yellow squash and zucchini.

+ Make delicious soups from a wide variety of vegetables.

Delicatessen choices

+ Select small amounts of sliced roast beef, turkey, or lean ham that is 97 or 98 percent fat-free.

+ Eat bacon sparingly, if at all.

+ Avoid hot dogs—even those made with turkey and chicken. They are high in fat.

Selecting dairy foods

+ Use plain nonfat yogurt as a substitute for sour cream.
+ Choose nonfat or low-fat cheeses, or cheese with less than five grams of fat per ounce such as Alpine Lace Swiss cheese, mozzarella, scamorza, ricotta, and nonfat cottage cheese.
+ Use fat-free milk.
+ Try buttermilk—it's low in fat.
+ Use only small amounts of margarine, preferably choosing the new nonfat varieties that have no trans-fatty acids; extra-virgin olive oil can be used instead of margarine.

The array of breads and cereals

+ Use whole-wheat and whole-grain breads (rye, oat bran, oat nut).
+ When selecting cereals, combine wheat bran and oat bran, choosing brands such as Kashi, All Bran, and Fiber One (eat one-third to one-half cup daily of these type cereals). When selecting a cereal made of oat bran alone, such as Quaker Oat Bran, eat one-third cup daily. Wheat helps to protect the colon; oat lowers cholesterol.
+ Be wary of granola-type cereals. Often they contain too much fat.

Surveying the meat counter

+ Avoid animal fat as much as possible, as well as organ meats such as liver and sweetbreads.
+ Use lean, trimmed cuts of meat—flank steaks, round steaks, sirloins, tenderloins, and ground sirloin, round, and chuck.
+ Eat pork sparingly. It is generally very high in fat; the tenderloin of pork is lowest in fat (26 percent); bacon is one of the highest (80 percent).
+ Choose *select* instead of *choice* or *prime* cuts of meat.
+ Limit or avoid ribs, corned beef, sausage, and bacon.

Fish and poultry choices

+ Choose fish from deep, cold-water regions. This includes salmon, tuna, mackerel, sea trout, herring, and cod.

+ Limit your intake of shrimp; use lobster and crab sparingly.

+ Use fresh ground turkey instead of ground beef.

+ Eat whole turkey or turkey breast steaks; they are excellent choices of meat.

+ When eating chicken, remember that half the calories in chicken are in the skin—discard the skin before cooking. To keep chicken moist during cooking, baste with olive oil.

Finding frozen foods

+ Choose frozen dinners with less than fifteen milligrams fat, less than four hundred calories, and less than eight hundred milligrams of sodium.

+ Buy frozen juice concentrates to make juice.

+ Use iced milk and nonfat frozen yogurt instead of ice cream.

+ For dessert, choose frozen juice bars and frozen fruit bars without added sugar.

Choosing fats, oils, and dressings

+ Use vegetable oil for cooking—the best choice is extra-virgin olive oil; canola oil is a good second choice.

+ Use olive oil for salads (it is the best choice), or prepare or purchase one of the wonderful no-oil dressings available now.

+ Use low-fat, no cholesterol vegetable spray (such as Pam) instead of oil or butter.

+ A butter substitute such as Butter Buds can be used on potatoes and other vegetables, or as a spread for breads and rolls.

+ Use fat-free mayonnaise.

+ Use diet dressings that contain less than ten calories per tablespoon.

+ Use low-fat or fat-free Italian dressings for salads and as a marinade for meat, poultry, and vegetables.

♦ Use seasoned vinegars, lemon juice, or herb and spice blends on vegetables and fish or chicken.

Packaged products

♦ Avoid palm, palm kernel, and coconut oils (read the labels before you buy).

♦ Eat unsalted pretzels sparingly for a low-fat snack.

♦ Because microwave popcorn is often high in fat (the wrong kind of fat) and salt, use air-popped popcorn instead.

♦ Eat potato chips sparingly. When you do purchase chip products, select the no-salt, fat-free choices available now.

♦ To lower cholesterol, choose from several types of dried beans that will lower cholesterol. These include great northern, pinto, kidney, and navy beans.

♦ Choose rice wisely—long-grain brown rice is a good choice.

♦ Buy cookies only if they contain *no* palm or coconut oil and have no more than three grams of fat per cookie; they are usually high in fat (read the labels). Try cookies made with fruit juices and no hydrogenated oils (found in the health food section).

What about canned foods?

♦ Avoid fruit punches and drinks; use 100 percent pure fruit juice.

♦ Select canned fish with edible bones such as salmon or sardines (watch the sodium levels in canned fish).

♦ Canned beans, peas, and corn are all good sources of vitamins, minerals, and fiber. However, they are not as nutritious as fresh—use them for convenience only when necessary.

EZEKIEL BREAD

The Bible cure actually recommends a particular bread to eat. Since it is described in Ezekiel, I have called it *Ezekiel bread*.

> Also take wheat, barley, beans, lentils, millet, and spelt, and put them into one vessel and make bread of them. (...לְךָ לְלֶחֶם
> וּפוֹל וַעֲדָשִׁים וְדֹחַן וְכֻסְּמִים וְנָתַתָּה אוֹתָם בִּכְלִי אֶחָד וְעָשִׂיתָ אוֹתָם
> (רְאֵה קַח־לְךָ חִטִּין וּשְׂעֹרִים.)
> —EZEKIEL 4:9, AMPC

In the text we see an amazing revelation from the Bible cure. Each specific food contained in the bread mentioned in Ezekiel 4:9 has particular benefits for our health and for preventing disease. Of course, God knew this, and He provided us this wonderful bread for our health and healing.

Here are just a few scientific findings about these food items:

+ *Wheat and spelt lower risk for heart disease.* Be sure you use whole wheat, including the bran and germ—not refined wheat. Whole wheat is an excellent source of B complex vitamins, phosphorus, iron, and vitamin E. The vitamin E in wheat helps the body reduce the production of free radicals (which cause LDL cholesterol to stick to artery walls), thus reducing the risk of heart disease. The fiber in wheat helps to reduce the risk of colon cancer.

+ *Barley also helps to lower your risk of heart disease.* Do your arteries a favor by eating both wheat and barley. Barley can help lower cholesterol, reduce the formation of blood clots, improve digestion, and reduce the risk of certain forms of cancer. It fights heart disease in two ways: The tocopherols in barley help to stop free radical oxidation, a process that makes LDL cholesterol (the dangerous type) stick to artery walls. They also help to prevent tiny blood clots from forming. Because barley is high in selenium and vitamin E, it helps protect and fight against cancer.

+ *Beans (pinto, lentils, kidney, great northern, and others) help lower cholesterol and are packed with soluble fiber.* They can also help to stabilize blood sugar levels, reduce the risk of breast and prostate cancers, and lower the risk of heart disease in people with diabetes.

+ *Millet and spelt can help to ease premenstrual discomfort and to speed healing in wounds.* Millet contains protein, which helps the body build and repair muscles, connective fibers, and other tissues.

Ezekiel bread can be purchased or made from the recipe below. (Find more healthy recipes in appendix B.)

Ezekiel Bread, a Recipe from the Old Testament*

2½ cups whole wheat
1½ cups whole rye
½ cup barley
¼ cup millet
¼ cup lentils
2 Tbsp. great northern beans (uncooked)
2 Tbsp. red kidney beans (uncooked)
2 Tbsp. pinto beans (uncooked)
2 cups lukewarm water, divided
½ cup plus 1 tsp. honey, divided
2 Tbsp. yeast
¼ cup extra-virgin olive oil

Measure and combine all the dry ingredients, except the yeast, in a large bowl. Put this mixture into a flour mill and grind. The flour should be the consistency of regular flour. Coarse flour may cause digestion problems. This makes eight cups of flour. Use four cups per batch of bread.

Measure four cups of flour into a large bowl. Store the remaining flour mixture in the freezer for future use.

Measure one cup lukewarm water (110–115 degrees) in a small mixing bowl. Add 1 teaspoon of the honey and the yeast, stir to dissolve the yeast, cover, and set aside, allowing the yeast to rise for five to ten minutes.

In a small mixing bowl combine the following: olive oil, ½ cup honey, and remaining cup of warm water. Mix well and add this to the flour mixture in the large bowl. Add the yeast to the bowl and stir until well mixed. The mixture should be the consistency of slightly "heavy" cornbread. Spread the mixture evenly in an 11 x 15-inch pan sprayed with no-cholesterol cooking oil. Let the mixture rise for one hour in a warm place. Bake at 375 degrees for approximately thirty minutes. Check for doneness. Bread should be the consistency of baked cornbread.

If a flour mill is not available for your use, Ezekiel flour can be ordered from a baking catalog or through a health food store. If such flours are used, however, the texture of the bread will be entirely different from the above recipe.

* This recipe has been adapted directly from Ezekiel 4:9.

SECTION THREE

NATURAL HEALTH SECRETS FOR CURING DISEASE

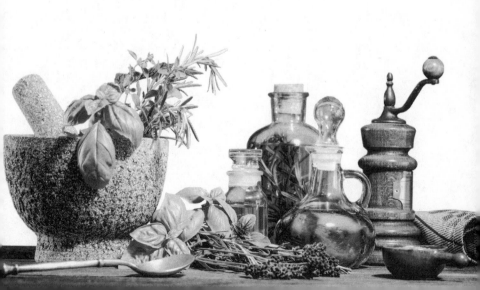

CHAPTER 8

BALANCE THE IMMUNE SYSTEM

Surely He shall deliver you from the snare of the fowler and from the perilous pestilence....No evil shall befall you, nor shall any plague come near your dwelling.

—PSALM 91:3, 10, NKJV

GOD PROMISES TO protect His people. Psalm 91 contains a beautiful description of the blessings of protection that God has made available to His children. Not only does God's protection shield us from our spiritual enemies, but also part of His blessing is protection from any *plagues* or *pestilence* that might try to come upon us. Plagues and pestilence signify disease, but God's children don't have to fear such contagion, for we are promised a satisfying, lengthy life. Take a moment to read the comforting promises God gives to us in several verses of this psalm:

> He who dwells in the shelter of the Most High shall abide under the shadow of the Almighty. I will say of the LORD, "He is my refuge and my fortress, my God in whom I trust." Surely He shall deliver you from the snare of the hunter and from the deadly pestilence....Because you have made the LORD, who is my refuge, even the Most High, your dwelling, there shall be no evil befall you, neither shall any plague come near your tent; for He shall give His angels charge over you to guard you in all your ways....Because he has set his love upon Me, therefore I will deliver him; I will set him on high, because he has known My name. He shall call upon Me, and I will answer him; I will be with him in trouble, and I will deliver him and honor him. With long life I will satisfy him and show him My salvation.

> —PSALM 91:1–3, 9–11, 14–16

PROTECTION FROM PLAGUES AND PESTILENCE

One way God chooses to protect us from disease is through the natural immune system that He built into our bodies. It is our "hedge of protection" between our bodies and the harmful bacteria and viruses that are present in the world. Because the Christian's body is, quite literally, the temple of the Holy Spirit (1 Cor. 6:19), how much more should we protect it from harm? By learning how our bodies function, as well as how to keep our immune systems balanced and working properly, we will be able to fight off the many diseases that are rampant in our world today and thus receive God's promise of a long and healthy life.

Unfortunately many people suffer from one or more diseases, the causes of which they really don't understand. The list of illnesses that spring from an imbalance in the immune system runs a virtual gamut of "plagues," including asthma, rheumatoid arthritis, moderate to severe allergies, inflammatory bowel disease (including Crohn's disease), Hodgkin's disease, leukemia, and even more dreaded forms of cancer.

How can you begin to implement God's promises of protection against plagues and pestilence into the daily world in which you live? You must begin to follow His commands for healthy eating patterns that will bring your immune system back into the balance He created it to have.

DISEASES OF THE IMMUNE SYSTEM

Diseases of the immune system fall into three primary categories:

+ Illnesses that result from an overactive immune system
+ Illnesses that result from an underactive immune system
+ Diseases that indicate the immune system has turned on the body and is attacking itself

To gain an understanding of what happens when things go awry in your immune system, first take a look at how it was designed to function.

The human body contains a vast array of various kinds of cells—white blood cells, lymphocytes, T cells, and natural killer cells—all designed to ward off any invasions of the body, especially those that would cause a catastrophic illness. Scientists call certain kinds of cells "natural killer cells" because their job is to hunt down and kill these foreign invaders that cause disease. One of these types of killer cells is called a *macrophage*, meaning "big eater." God created this cell to devour, much like Pac-Man in the old video arcade game, any dangerous or foreign substances that enter the body.

Proper functioning of the T cells is very important because they act as the "commanders of the army," directing the macrophages into battle. God's promise in Psalm 91 is realized through the macrophages already present in your own body. Every time you successfully fight off a cold, for example, you can thank God for His Word and that His promises are always true—your immune system has turned away yet another plague from your dwelling place—and His!

So many times when people think of diseases of the immune system, they jump to the conclusion that these diseases occur when the immune system has somehow been compromised or knocked out altogether. A classic example of this would be the AIDS virus, which results in the immune system becoming deficient and underactive, leaving the person vulnerable to any number of contagious and deadly diseases. AIDS itself is not what kills a person; the diseases to which the person is helplessly exposed strike the fatal blow because of an underactive immune system.

However, an underactive immune system is not the only way the body becomes compromised. If the body's immune system becomes *overactive*, serious problems can also occur, and if it reaches the point where the body's defenses begin to *attack itself*, a whole new category of illnesses, referred to as *autoimmune disorders*, is the result. A closer look at these three problems will help you know how to walk toward healing.

Underactive immune system

When the immune system is no longer capable of stopping an attack, the person becomes vulnerable to all types of terrible "plagues." If you are someone who frequently catches colds or has difficulty getting over them, your immune system could be compromised in some way. Respiratory infections, viral infections—including the Zika virus that is causing such a stir—and, of course, the ultimate failure of the immune system—cancer—belong in this first category of illnesses.

Did you know that every one of us develops a form of cancer once or twice a week throughout our entire lives? A "cancerous" cell is simply a cell that has gone astray—it begins to divide abnormally on its own until it has divided enough times to get out of control. Our immune systems are designed to recognize those cells as soon as an abnormal division takes place. Then our T cells lead our macrophages ("big eaters") into battle to kill and eat up the cancer before it progresses. The cancers that go on to cause problems and eventually kill people are indicative of a failure of the immune system to catch the problem in time.

Overactive immune system

Many people believe that the more active their immune system is, the better off they are, but that is not the case. Sometimes the body becomes so "paranoid" about potential invasion that it begins to recognize harmless substances as foreign invaders to be attacked, sometimes with great fervor. Moderate or severe allergies are classic examples of this phenomenon. When something harmless, such as a miniscule dust mite or piece of pollen, is breathed in, the immune system, sensing grave danger, begins to send a flood of histamine on the attack to squeeze liquid out of the cells and flush the foreign particle out of the system. This is what causes the sneezing, wheezing, coughing, and runny eyes and nose that make people miserable.

Other diseases that demonstrate this overactivity include asthma—in which the body's reaction is wheezing and shortness of breath—and chronic fatigue syndrome or fibromyalgia—in which the body responds with fatigue and a total lack of energy.

Autoimmune disorders

Sometimes the body's immune system goes totally haywire, and instead of attacking a foreign invader, it begins to attack the body itself. In multiple sclerosis, for example, the body literally attacks the myelin sheath that lines the nerve endings. In inflammatory bowel disease, including Crohn's disease and ileitis, the body attacks its own lower digestive tract. Other diseases in this category include lupus, rheumatoid arthritis, and scleroderma.

Interestingly, autoimmune diseases are much more common among women than they are among men, possibly due to a hormonal relationship of which we are not yet fully aware.

WE'VE MISSED THE ROOT CAUSE

Traditional medicine typically attempts to treat these diseases individually by coming up with a new antibiotic to combat viruses, new nasal sprays to alleviate allergy symptoms, or new treatments to shrink cancerous tumors. While these treatments have their place, none of them are dealing with the root cause: an immune system that is out of balance.

How many times have you been treated for a recurring virus with another round of antibiotics? That has become such a pat answer for most infections that it doesn't even occur to some doctors that it might not be the best solution. Antibiotics can be harmful to our bodies because they kill not only the "bad" bacteria but also the "good" bacteria, or flora, in our intestines that help promote healthy immune system function.

The times in which we live today are dangerous ones, as the threat of bioterrorism has become increasingly real in the last several years. The fear used to be that some diseases such as smallpox might accidentally reappear, but now the fear is that they will be released on the world intentionally. In addition, new strains of viruses that have never before been reported in the United States are now on the rise, such as Zika and Ebola.

In the development of "cures" for these diseases, traditional medicine inadvertently can create as much harm as good: for years the drug methicillin was used to kill off the deadly *Staphylococcus* bacteria, but now much of these bacteria have become resistant to the drug. What are we to do? How can we protect ourselves? It is not time to become hopeless or to lose heart. It is time to remember the promises of Psalm 91—God has not left us defenseless.

In these last days God is beginning to bring awareness to the medical community of the root cause of many of the diseases that plague millions of Americans. Giving proper attention to the immune system can bring the answer to health we are searching for. The answer does not necessarily lie in stimulating or "revving up" the immune systems of patients across the board. Although there are cases in which its ability to recognize and wipe out disease needs to be increased, other cases require a *decrease* in immune system function. When people take certain products inappropriately to enhance their immunity or overuse antibiotics to try to prevent infections, they run the risk of developing other serious problems, such as asthma and allergies or, even worse, some of the devastating autoimmune disorders.

Putting "Glasses" on the Immune System

The key, as it is with many things in God's kingdom, is *balance*. Our goal must be to restore our immune system to a healthy balance, in which it responds correctly to dangerous situations but lets harmless particles through without a fuss.

I like to describe the restoration of this balance as *putting glasses on the immune system*. For example, if you have poor vision, you are unable to recognize things clearly. When someone knocks on your door, you may squint through the peephole, see someone who looks like your best friend, and then swing open the door—only to welcome an intruder. Or if you see someone on the street who looks like an enemy, you may try to defend yourself, not realizing that it is a friend you're attacking.

Perhaps that seems like an extreme example, but that is what the immune system is doing in many of these diseases. Like a person suffering with poor vision, it has lost the ability to distinguish between friend and foe. So what we want to do is put glasses on the immune system—to restore its vision and its ability to recognize true danger and respond appropriately. The key to that process is balance.

NUTRIENTS THAT PROTECT AND RESTORE PROPER IMMUNE SYSTEM FUNCTION

A natural decline in immune system function takes place in every person as they age, beginning as early as the thirties, due to a deficiency in certain nutrients throughout life. That is why every person, regardless of whether or not they are demonstrating symptoms of any of these diseases, should be protecting their immune systems with nutritional supplements. I have listed below the common nutrients along with proper dosages to take to ensure a healthy immune system throughout your life span.

Vitamin E

I recommend 800 international units daily to protect the immune system.

Tocotrienols

The tocotrienols are "cousins" of vitamin E and are essential for vitamin E to work properly. I recommend 105 milligrams of tocotrienols daily.

Vitamin C

Vitamin C is critical for lymphocyte function, which is why it is good to drink orange juice when you have a cold. I recommend 2 grams of vitamin C (2,000 milligrams) per day.

Zinc

To simply protect the immune system, I recommend 15 milligrams per day. Use caution, however, when taking zinc, as it affects the absorption of copper in the body. It would be best to take zinc in the form of a multivitamin that also supplements copper, for if you increase your zinc intake without also increasing copper, you may become copper deficient. And because copper is necessary for white blood cell function, any deficiencies will adversely affect the immune system—the very opposite of the effect you originally intended to achieve!

Additionally, too much zinc in the system will interfere with immune system function, so be sure to avoid the misconception that "more is better." That is not always the case! Please take only the dosages that are recommended, and you will avoid a host of unnecessary problems.

Beta-carotene

Beta-carotene is transformed by the body into vitamin A, known to strengthen the immune system. Beta-carotene is preferable to taking higher doses of vitamin A, which can affect liver function. The body will take the beta-carotene it receives and manufacture only the vitamin A that it needs from that. I recommend 20,000 international units a day.

Selenium

Selenium is a mineral that has been shown to be critical to the immune system by stimulating our "natural killer" cells that attack harmful viruses or cancers. It also balances the immune system to work more effectively. One study done over a period of ten years looked at the immune systems of thirteen hundred people who took 200 micrograms of selenium a day. The rates of cancer development (every type of cancer) in this group of people dropped 40 percent, and the rates of lung, prostate, and colon cancer specifically were reduced by 50 percent![1] For this reason, I recommend 200 micrograms daily.

Author's note

If you are facing one of the diseases we listed that is related to a malfunctioning immune system, it is necessary to increase the dosages of the nutrients listed below to the given levels:

+ *Vitamin E:* Increase to 1,000 international units daily.
+ *Tocotrienols:* Continue taking 105 milligrams per day.
+ *Vitamin C:* Increase to 2,500 milligrams per day (taken with food).
+ *Zinc:* Increase (cautiously) to 25 milligrams per day. Be sure to increase your copper intake as well to maintain a healthy balance.
+ *Beta-carotene:* Increase to 25,000 international units per day.
+ *Selenium:* Increase to 320 micrograms per day.

HERBAL PREPARATIONS TO ENHANCE THE IMMUNE SYSTEM

Numerous herbs have been found within God's plant kingdom that restore balance to the immune system. Most modern prescriptions that man has devised for immune system function *either* slow down *or* stimulate the immune system; they do not work to balance it. God's natural substances do both, slowing and stimulating as needed; His purpose is balance in all things. The natural herbs listed below are God's provision for enhancing the immune system.

Pomegranate seed

Pomegranates have been around at least since biblical times. Studies from Israel are now reporting that pomegranate extract triggers a self-destruction mechanism in breast cancer cells. It is the first time that a common ingredient has been found to stimulate the immune system to attack cancer in the body.[2] My recommendation is 50 milligrams per day.

Elderberry

Another study from researchers in Israel examined the effect of elderberry on common viral influenzas. Elderberry performed two functions: it directly inhibited the virus itself, and it stimulated the immune system to attack the virus more vigorously. The effect was that flu symptoms were reduced by 50 percent.[3] A later study also offered encouraging results. Sixty individuals exhibiting flu-like symptoms were in the study; those given elderberry recovered four days sooner, on average, than those who received a placebo.[4] I recommend common elderberry in the extract form, 100 milligrams a day.

Astragalus

Astragalus promotes an increase in the number of T cells ("commanders of the army") in the body, boosting resistance to infection and, even more importantly, countering the age-related decline that all of us see in our immune systems. As we get older, our T cell counts decline, most commonly due to poor dietary habits and the polluted environment, but astragalus overcomes that decline and can restore the immune system to that of a twenty-year-old. I recommend 100 milligrams a day.

Beta 1,3 glucans

Beta 1,3 glucans are polysaccharide compounds, a type of complex carbohydrate commonly found in the cell walls of baker's yeast and also found in a slightly different form in mushrooms. Like some of the other substances I have mentioned, beta glucans stimulate a weakened immune system but will not overstimulate it (unlike many prescription medications do). Beta glucans strengthen the macrophage ("big eaters") function and have been shown to significantly reduce the risk of postoperative infections. The daily recommended dose is 25 milligrams per day.

Mushrooms

Mushrooms promote healthy immune systems because they contain beta 1,3 glucans. There are three main classifications of mushrooms, each of which originated in Asia, all having slightly different healing properties. The *maitake* mushroom has been called the "king of the mushrooms." According to one study performed in China, the maitake mushroom both inhibited cancerous tumors from forming and killed cancer cells associated with lung, stomach, and liver cancer by stimulating the T cells and the macrophages.[5] The *reishi* mushroom has been shown effective in the treatment of allergies and asthma by bringing an overstimulated immune system back into balance and inhibiting the release of histamine against harmless agents. The *shiitake* mushroom contains an unusual compound called lentinan, which is extremely potent in balancing the immune system and in the prevention of cancer.

Garlic

Garlic is used for many different reasons as it affects multiple body systems. It has been found to alter cholesterol levels and enhance the cardiovascular system in addition to its benefits to the immune system. There are thirty different cancer-fighting compounds in garlic alone.

If you are wondering about how to implement all of these nutrients into your diet in a tasty way, please try the recipe for "Cancer-Fighting Lentil Soup" that my wife, Linda, has developed; it is delicious. (See appendix B.) In addition to making changes in your diet to consume natural nutrients, I also recommend that you supply your body with the supplements we have discussed that will restore balance to your immune system.

THE SYNERGISTIC EFFECT

You will see the greatest effect in the restoration of your immune system when you combine these supplemental nutrients and common herbs and incorporate them into a more natural, healthy diet. They will work together in your body to balance your immune system so that it can provide resistance against viruses, harmful bacteria, and cancer, as well as preventing it from attacking harmless substances or even your own body.

If you have any of the diseases that have been discussed in this chapter, let me encourage you to begin a three-pronged attack against them:

+ *Pray* that God would put "glasses" on your immune system so that it will recognize and attack only the things it was intended to attack.

+ *Read the Word.* Begin to speak Psalm 91 over your life, declaring the promises for protection from plagues and pestilence and for a long and satisfying life.

+ *Supplement.* Begin a regimen of supplementing your healthy diet with these nutrients and herbs and with other protocol from advice you receive in this book for a healthy lifestyle.

ESSENTIAL NUTRIENTS FOR A BALANCED IMMUNE SYSTEM			
Nutrient	**Effect**	**Daily Dosage**	**Treatment Dosage**
Astragalus root powder	Herb widely used in traditional Chinese medicine to provide immune support	50 mg	100 mg
Beta glucan	Naturally derived plant substance known to boost immune function	25 mg	25 mg
Elderberry fruit powder	Herb traditionally used to support healthy respiratory and immune function	50 mg	100 mg
Garlic bulb extract	Herb widely used as a natural antimicrobial and immune enhancer	100 mg	100 mg
Maitake mushroom	Herb traditionally used as an aid to healthy immune and liver function	25 mg	25 mg
Pomegranate fruit extract	Herbal extract that is rich in antioxidant flavonoids	25 mg	50 mg
Reishi mushroom	Herb that contains a broad spectrum of antioxidant, detoxifying, and immunomodulating substances	5 mg	5 mg

ESSENTIAL NUTRIENTS FOR A BALANCED IMMUNE SYSTEM			
Nutrient	**Effect**	**Daily Dosage**	**Treatment Dosage**
Selenium	Essential mineral that enhances many aspects of immune function and helps protect against a number of chronic diseases	200 mcg	320 mcg
Shiitake mushroom	Herb rich in immunomodulating substances that has been widely used in China and Japan for its immune-enhancing effects	5 mg	5 mg
Mixed tocotrienol complex	Important component of vitamin E with potent antioxidant activity	105 mg	105 mg
Beta-carotene	Essential vitamin that plays an important role in maintaining a healthy immune system	20,000 IU	25,000 IU
Vitamin C	Essential vitamin that enhances the body's natural resistance to invasion by harmful microorganisms	2,000 mg	2,500 mg
Zinc	Essential mineral that boosts immune function and has been shown in studies to reduce the duration and severity of respiratory infections	15 mg	25 mg
Vitamin E	Essential vitamin that protects the immune system	800 IU	1,000 IU

CHAPTER 9

DIABETES: STARVING IN THE LAND OF PLENTY

Thus says the LORD, the God of David your father: I have heard your prayer; I have seen your tears. I will heal you.

—2 KINGS 20:5

FATIGUE. BLINDNESS. DISFIGUREMENT due to amputations. One devastating disease that affects millions of people is capable of wreaking havoc in the health and lives of those people upon whom it preys. You may not be aware that what actually occurs in a diabetic's body is starvation in the land of plenty. Even in the presence of nutrients, the cells of the body are unable to absorb what they need, resulting in multiple horrific symptoms.

Isn't it just like the devil to try to steal the provisions that God gives us, right from under our noses? In diabetes he is literally "dangling a carrot" of glucose within millimeters of the cell wall, but because of the disease, the much-needed blood sugar is still just out of reach.

Diabetes is a disease that is reaching epidemic proportions in our society today. According to the Centers for Disease Control, approximately 29.1 million Americans suffer from the effects of diabetes, but 27 percent of these—about 8.1 million people—don't even know that they have it![1]

Over four thousand new cases of diabetes are diagnosed—not every month, not every week—but *every day*.[2] Right now, diabetes has cost the American people over $245 billion.[3] The rate of diabetes has doubled in the general population in the last thirty years.[4] Doctors and researchers used to call type 2 diabetes "adult-onset diabetes" because it very rarely struck anyone younger than the age of forty-five. But now our definition is beginning to change because people as young as teenagers are developing glucose intolerance, which results in type 2 diabetes by the time they reach their twenties.

Why has diabetes become such an epidemic? Probably the biggest factor involved is the sedentary lifestyle of most Americans, which leads to weight gain. Over half of all Americans are now considered to be overweight, and this "extra baggage" is very harmful to their health. Specifically, being overweight causes the body to be less sensitive to the insulin it produces. In addition, the typical diet—high in saturated fats and sugars—that Americans consume is very conducive to the development of diabetes.

WHAT IS DIABETES?

When a person eats a meal, the nutrients from the food are absorbed and enter the bloodstream to be carried to the cells of the body. *Glucose*, or blood sugar, is the primary molecule derived from food that passes through the walls of the blood vessels to reach the *receptor cells* of the muscles, nerves, or other organs that need the blood sugar to function properly. The *pancreas* is the organ of the body that produces *insulin*, the primary substance that helps to transport the blood sugar into the cells of the body. As insulin is secreted by the pancreas into the bloodstream, the glucose levels in the blood are lowered as the blood sugar begins to pass through the walls of the blood vessels and into the receptor cells, which are waiting for nutrition.

Most people, following a fast, will have a glucose level of between 70 and 110—a normal level of glucose in the blood. But a diabetic's glucose level could reach 300. The unfortunate irony of this disease, however, is that despite the huge amount of sugar in the bloodstream, just out of reach of the receptor cells, the body is actually starving to death. Why? Because of something called *insulin resistance*.

Insulin resistance occurs because receptor cells that have been exposed to too much insulin become desensitized and are no longer able to absorb nutrients into the cells. In the beginning stages of diabetes, the pancreas still secretes normal levels of insulin, but as blood sugar rises, the body signals the pancreas to produce more insulin in order to get rid of the glut of sugar that is backing up in the bloodstream. The body is literally crying out, "More insulin over here, please!" since insulin is what transports sugar out of the blood into the cells.

Unfortunately, insulin levels that are either too high or too low will become a poison to the body. If insulin levels are too low, the body will starve because insulin is necessary for the absorption of nutrients. But when the pancreas begins to secrete more and more insulin into the bloodstream, the walls of the blood vessels are literally attacked with the substance. When this occurs in the coronary arteries or the vessels near the brain, risks of heart attack or stroke increase dramatically. In fact, many of my diabetic patients eventually die of a heart attack, a statistic that is corroborated by medical organizations. Sixty-eight percent of diabetics over the age of 65 die because of heart disease, and another 16 percent die because of a stroke.[5]

Spikes in insulin levels also decrease the sensitivity of the receptors to the point that they no longer function properly and the cells can no longer absorb the nutrients that are "right outside of their grasp." Eventually the pancreas wears itself out by overproducing so much insulin, and the person is forced to begin *insulin therapy*. Because their bodies no longer produce their own insulin, these people have to inject themselves with the insulin their body needs.

Many times this problem of insulin resistance is compounded by our insatiable consumption of sugary junk foods. What exactly happens when you eat that box of sugar doughnuts or indulge in that midafternoon Snickers bar? Shortly after the taste has faded from your mouth, your blood glucose level suddenly spikes as the sugar from the candy or the doughnut enters your bloodstream. Your body reacts by sending in a flux of insulin to counteract the glucose. These spikes in the insulin level are what decrease receptor sensitivity and create the insulin resistance. With certain types of sugar and junk food, the levels will first spike very high and then plummet very low, causing you to feel a burst of energy followed by fatigue and sluggishness.

The human body is designed to function best when there are gradual rises and declines in the glucose levels of the bloodstream. But our modern lifestyle, full of fast food that is overprocessed and sadly lacking in nutrition, serves to promote the development of diseases such as diabetes. In other words, the food we eat is not only lacking in needed nutrition, but it is also killing us.

SYMPTOMS OF DIABETES

The following common symptoms of diabetes should be carefully noted, especially since diabetes consistently goes undiagnosed in people until it has progressed to dangerous phases:

+ *Increased thirst.* When the body is facing an unusual amount of glucose in the bloodstream, it calls upon the kidneys to help get rid of the oversupply. This increases the need for fluid, hence, increased thirst. Accompanying this symptom is *increased urination*, the kidneys' attempt to flush the bloodstream of the excess glucose.

+ *Fatigue.* As the disease progresses, although there is more than adequate nutrition in the blood, the cells are not receiving it due to insulin resistance, as I explained. For this reason most diabetics complain of feeling totally exhausted. Ironically they have the highest fuel supply in their bloodstream (300–400 glucose levels), but their cells are literally starving to death.

+ *Weight loss.* As the body continues to starve, it will begin to feed on its stores of fat and muscle, and the person will begin to lose weight.

+ *Blurred vision.* As sugar levels in the blood continue to rise, the blood vessels in the eyes will begin to be adversely affected. If left unchecked, diabetes will lead to partial or complete *blindness.* In fact, diabetes is one of the leading causes of blindness.[6]

+ *Neuropathy.* Every nerve in the body is connected to a blood vessel in order to receive life-giving nutrients, which means that every nerve in the body is affected by the high glucose levels of diabetes. As the disease progresses, the person will notice tingling in the extremities as nerves become damaged, a condition known as neuropathy. Advanced *peripheral neuropathy* affects extremities, leading to increased lack of feeling in the arms and legs and potentially dangerous sores, which go unnoticed by the person, leading to infections or even gangrene. Often amputation becomes the necessary drastic measure that must be taken to save the patient's life. Advanced *autonomic neuropathy* affects internal organs of the body, such as nerves to the stomach, making the patient unable to digest food properly, or nerves to the male genitalia, making the person impotent.

+ *Kidney failure.* Finally, because the kidneys work so hard to remove excess glucose from the blood, the incidence of renal disease, kidney failure, and dialysis increase dramatically in the diabetic population.

DIAGNOSING DIABETES

I cannot emphasize enough how important it is for you, if you are experiencing any of these symptoms, to go to your doctor right away to have your blood sugar levels tested. It is easy to overlook the symptoms and pretend that nothing is wrong. A few years ago I saw a patient who thought he had found a new way to lose weight by drinking lots of water. He did not realize that both his weight loss and his thirst were classic symptoms of diabetes. When I performed a blood test on him, we discovered that his glucose level was over 350!

Be aware of the wiles of the devil; he would love to take out as many members of the body of Christ as he can with this deadly disease. If you have any of the symptoms of diabetes, be sure to consult with your physician immediately. He can perform simple tests to determine whether you are struggling with diabetes.

Glycosylated hemoglobin test

This test is more simply known as the Hemoglobin A1c. Its advantage over several others is that it averages a person's blood sugar levels over a time period of three months instead of just taking a random sampling here and there. This is important because a true diabetic's numbers can vary drastically from day to day.

The goal of the A1c test is one simple number: keep the A1c under 6.4, and you will be all right.

Glucose tolerance test (GTT)

This test requires the patient to take 75 grams of glucose and have their blood levels tested two hours later. Problems occur when this number reaches the level of 150 to 200.

Fasting blood sugar test

If after a twelve-hour fast a patient's blood sugar level reaches 126 or higher on two or more different days, by definition the patient is diagnosed as having diabetes.

CONVENTIONAL TREATMENTS FOR DIABETES

Many Christians resist the idea of taking medication for a disease or illness, but if you need to be on a prescription medicine or insulin treatment for diabetes, it may save your life. There are several natural treatments for the disease, which I will discuss later in this chapter. But most of the prescription drugs that are available for diabetes are much more effective at lowering the patient's blood sugar levels *quickly* and *predictably*.

If you are just discovering that you are a diabetic, chances are that you need to lower your glucose levels, and you need to lower them *fast*. Often the best plan, the plan that God guides many people to take, is to begin to take the prescription medicine immediately, but also to begin taking natural supplements at the same time. Many times when the glucose levels are stabilized, the patient can begin to back off some of the prescriptions. But I cannot emphasize enough that *any changes that you make must be made under a doctor's supervision and while your blood levels are being monitored.* Diabetes is a dangerous disease; don't allow the enemy to get a foothold in your life by ignoring wisdom and prudence. Allow your doctor to be an instrument of God's healing in your life.

Medications to treat diabetes have classically addressed the diminishing levels of insulin in the bloodstream. Glucotrol is one among several of these drugs that stimulate the pancreas to secrete more insulin, but this is not an ideal solution to the problem. Certainly, diabetics whose insulin levels are too low will either need a way to produce more insulin within their own bodies or to receive shots of insulin that are injected directly into their bloodstream. However, increasing insulin levels simply to counteract increasing glucose levels in the blood does not address the root of the problem, and, as I mentioned before, too much insulin is very harmful to the body.

Another class of drugs used to treat diabetes actually reduces the insulin resistance of the cells. Remember, insulin resistance occurs when cell receptors that have been exposed to too much insulin become desensitized and are no longer able to absorb nutrients from the bloodstream into the cells. Doctors are beginning to realize that if a patient's pancreas is still able to produce a normal level of insulin, perhaps a better strategy for treatment would be to cause the receptor cells to become more sensitive to the insulin that is already available.

A third class of prescription drugs is available for the treatment of diabetes. These drugs affect the breakdown of carbohydrates in the system, slowing them down, which in turn prevents the extreme glucose spikes in the bloodstream. Both glucose and insulin levels remain steady, and diabetic symptoms are brought under control.

NATURAL NUTRIENTS TO PREVENT
OR REVERSE DIABETES

I am so thankful to God that He has provided natural resources for healing. Many substances available in the plant and animal kingdoms very nearly duplicate the same effects of prescription medications used to treat diabetes. If you have diabetes, or if diabetes runs in your family, begin taking these nutrients *now* to begin slowing the progression of your disease or, better still, prevent or reverse it.

Chromium

Chromium is a natural trace mineral that should be present in our daily diets, but the majority of Americans are chromium deficient. Most of us consume only 30 micrograms of chromium a day, when we need 200 micrograms daily.

In the treatment of diabetes, chromium actually increases the effectiveness of insulin. That is, in the presence of chromium, the insulin produced in the pancreas actually does a better job of moving the glucose through the blood vessels and to the receptor cells.

Chromium can be found naturally in brewer's yeast, which is available at your local health food store. However, that may still not give you a sufficient amount daily. I recommend a chromium supplement of 300 micrograms a day for the *prevention* of diabetes and 800 to 1,000 micrograms a day for the *treatment* of the disease.

Vanadium

The trace element vanadium is also effective in enhancing the effect of the insulin already present in the body. Vanadium itself has insulin-like properties that cause blood sugar levels to drop. The same dosage of 300 micrograms daily is recommended for both preventive and treatment purposes.

Biotin

Biotin, one of the B vitamins, operates in much the same way as the third class of prescription medicines we discussed previously: it enhances the metabolism or the breakdown of carbohydrates, reducing the number of glucose spikes in the bloodstream. The ideal dosage for biotin is also 300 micrograms daily.

Niacin

Niacin performs the same function as biotin; that is, it increases carbohydrate metabolism. The dosage of niacin should be carefully monitored and kept to a maximum of 100 milligrams daily; this should help to prevent any adverse effects to the liver.

Magnesium

Many Americans are deficient in magnesium; the recommended daily dosage is 400 milligrams per day. Magnesium has numerous beneficial effects in the treatment of diabetes. First of all, it causes an increase in the excretion of glucose in the urine, thus helping to alleviate some of the excess blood sugars that a diabetic experiences. Magnesium, like biotin and niacin, also improves carbohydrate metabolism. And finally, magnesium increases the cellular sensitivity to insulin, diminishing insulin resistance, which is the greatest problem the majority of diabetics face.

Zinc

Again, most of our diets are deficient in the levels of zinc that we need. A 15-milligram daily dose is needed for the prevention and treatment of diabetes, but this is another nutrient that should be approached with caution. Some people think that if 15 milligrams are good, then ten times that would be even better. That is incorrect! Too much zinc will adversely affect the metabolism of both glucose and insulin, so please be sure to take only 15 milligrams per day.

Omega-3 fatty acids

God's provision made nutrients available to us in both the plant and animal kingdoms. The omega-3 fatty acids are found in the animal kingdom in the fatty fishes such as salmon, cod, mackerel, and herring. These fatty acids have been shown both to improve glucose breakdown and to decrease the body's resistance to insulin.

HERBAL PREPARATIONS TO COMBAT DIABETES

In addition to the seven essential nutrients listed above, there are four herbal preparations that are effective in combating diabetes and in controlling some of its complications. When used together, these nutrients and herbs have a *synergistic* effect, working together to become even more effective in bringing health to your body.

Fenugreek

Fenugreek, another herb with an unusual name, has been shown in studies to help control type 2 diabetes under the proper conditions. A 2009 article published in the *International Journal for Vitamin and Nutrition Research* showed that fenugreek added to hot water can help control diabetes.[7] Fenugreek is a plant that grows in parts of Europe and Asia. In fact, it is a regular part of the diet in India. It works differently in that it slows the absorption of sugar in the patient's gastrointestinal tract, thus lowering the glucose levels that reach the bloodstream. Fenugreek is the fiber portion of a certain herbal seed. It should be taken at a dosage of 15 to 25 grams per day.

Gymnema

This important herb with an unusual name is from a woody plant that grows in India and in the Far East. It has been used for centuries in the treatment of diabetes. Numerous benefits can be derived from the consumption of gymnema: it decreases blood sugar levels; it decreases insulin requirements; it regenerates the beta cells of the pancreas and allows them to produce more insulin; and it aids the glucose in crossing the blood vessel wall to reach nutritionally deprived cells.

Many patients have been able to reduce or phase out their prescription medications after a regimen of gymnema. It is now sold at health food stores and should be taken in a dosage of 400 milligrams per day.

Cinnamon

New research is showing that cinnamon supplements can help those with insulin resistance and diabetes. Four separate studies showed the benefits of supplementing with cinnamon. This includes studies showing benefits for those with diabetes and metabolic syndrome.[8] In a study on cinnamon supplements and hyperglycemic patients, patients showed a lower blood sugar level after fasting and after a meal if they took cinnamon rather than a placebo.[9] I recommend taking 1,000 milligrams of cinnamon per day to help control blood sugar levels.

Bitter melon

Bitter melon, like gymnema, has the effect of increasing glucose uptake (absorption) into the cells. It comes in an extract form and should be taken at a dose of 400 milligrams once a day.

Bilberry

Bilberry, or bilberry extract, prevents capillaries and blood vessels from leaking, a common problem among diabetics. Two hundred milligrams per day is the recommended dosage.

COUNTERACTING COMPLICATIONS OF DIABETES

Perhaps the most frightening aspect of diabetes lies in the numerous harrowing complications that could potentially occur: blindness, heart attacks, strokes, disfigurement or even amputation of the extremities, along with damage to internal organs. These complications may at first seem to be diverse, but they all stem from the same general problem: *neuropathy*. (See the explanation of *neuropathy* under "Symptoms of Diabetes" earlier in this chapter.) There are three important natural substances that can help prevent serious complications of diabetes.

Alpha lipoic acid

Alpha lipoic acid is produced in very small amounts in the human body, which is why it is not classified as a vitamin per se. When taken at a supplemental dose of 50 milligrams per day, it improves the metabolism of sugar, increases muscular energy, regenerates other powerful antioxidants such as vitamins C, E, and glutathione, and it protects against the possibility of neuropathy. However, if you are already suffering the effects of neuropathy, the suggested dose increases to 600 to 800 milligrams per day, depending on the severity of your symptoms. The good news is that alpha lipoic acid has no known side effects.

Gamma-linolenic acid (GLA)

GLA is an essential fatty acid, a cousin of the omega-3 fish oils, which we have already discussed. The dosage for diabetes prevention is 90 milligrams per day and for treatment is 400 to 500 milligrams per day.

Water-soluble B vitamins

Water-soluble B vitamins, including B_1, B_6, B_{12}, inositol, and B_5, increase nerve sheath conduction. When this takes place in the brain, the result is improved memory function, but the benefits can be reaped throughout the body. Water-soluble B vitamins nourish the nerves and supply damaged nerves with blood, preventing infection and gangrene in extremities as well as other complications.

DAILY REGIMEN TO PREVENT DIABETES

Neither my wife nor I have diabetes, but we do certain things every day to ensure that we never contract this deadly disease. I have listed below the six most important prevention techniques for diabetes. These techniques take self-discipline to implement in your life, but the results are worth the effort.

1. Take the three most important minerals daily.

These include the daily dosages of chromium, vanadium, and magnesium. Because so many of our diets are deficient in these minerals, I recommend taking them in supplement form. These three will make your own body's insulin more effective and decrease your cells' insulin resistance.

2. Take the daily dose of the antioxidants alpha lipoic acid and lycopene.

Alpha lipoic acid and lycopene are the most powerful antioxidants against the effects of diabetes. By taking a supplement of just 200 milligrams a day of alpha lipoic acid and 1,000 micrograms a day of lycopene, your blood insulin levels can be decreased significantly.

3. Take the essential fatty acids, including fish oil and GLA.

Omega-3 fatty acids (fish oil) and GLA are effective in preventing diabetes by improving glucose tolerance.

4. Watch your diet.

Cut back on the sugary junk food that causes your glucose levels to spike and then plummet. Adding the following nutrients to your diet will help immensely:

- Two servings a day of a whole-grain food product (dark rice; dark, crunchy bread; or a grainy cereal) will decrease the risk of diabetes by 33 percent.[10] One of the best cereals we have found for this purpose is called Bran Buds, made by Kellogg's.

- Psyllium is a fiber extract from the husk of the plantago plant, which can also be found in Bran Buds. It has been found to decrease blood sugar levels by 11 percent in people who consumed 2 tablespoons per day. In these same people it decreased the post-meal sugar levels (the dangerous glucose spikes) by 20 percent.[11]

- In addition to the chromium supplements you should already be taking, it's a good idea to add to your diet foods that are high in chromium. These include mushrooms, almonds, and prunes.

- Other foods that can prevent diabetes include onions, which contain diphenylamine, a compound that can decrease blood sugar levels as effectively as a prescription drug; cinnamon, which lowers blood sugar and increases cellular sensitivity to insulin; and beans, which slow the rise of glucose in the bloodstream. Who would have thought that such common foods, which most of us already have in our pantries, can help prevent one of the most deadly diseases in our society?

5. Exercise.

Check with your doctor before beginning any exercise program, but make sure that you work some form of regular exercise—whether it be walking, jogging, or playing tennis—into your lifestyle. Regular exercise can dramatically reduce the risk of diabetes.

6. Lose weight.

If you regularly follow steps one through five, you will lose weight as well. Obesity is a growing problem in America. Dropping the pounds will greatly decrease your risk for diabetes.

ESSENTIAL NUTRIENTS TO MAINTAIN HEALTHY GLUCOSE LEVELS			
Nutrient	**Effect**	**Preventive Dosage**	**Treatment Dosage**
Alpha lipoic acid	Improves sugar metabolism; regulates other antioxidants	200 mg	600–800 mg
Bitter melon fruit extract	Herb shown in both human and animal studies to have a beneficial effect on blood glucose levels[12]	400 mg	600 mg
Bilberry leaf extract	Herb used in traditional folk medicine to treat diabetes and its complications	200 mg	200 mg
Chromium	Essential trace mineral that plays a role in glucose regulation and helps increase the effectiveness of insulin	300 mcg	800–1,000 mcg
Fenugreek	Soluble fiber that slows the absorption of sugars from the intestinal tract; binds toxins; helps regulate cholesterol levels	15–25 g	15–25 g

ESSENTIAL NUTRIENTS TO MAINTAIN HEALTHY GLUCOSE LEVELS			
Nutrient	**Effect**	**Preventive Dosage**	**Treatment Dosage**
Gymnema leaf extract	Unique herb from India that has been shown to lower insulin requirements in clinical studies, possibly by helping to regenerate the insulin-producing cells of the pancreas[13]	400 mg	400 mg
Magnesium	Essential mineral needed for proper insulin function; often deficient in diabetics	400 mg	400 mg
Vanadium	Trace mineral known to support insulin function and improve glucose utilization	300 mcg	300 mcg
Biotin	B vitamin that enhances the metabolism of carbohydrates	300 mcg	300 mcg
Niacin	Vitamin that enhances the metabolism of carbohydrates	100 mg	100 mg
Gamma-linolenic acid	Improves glucose breakdown and decreases resistance to insulin	90 mg	90 mg
Cinnamon	Lowers blood sugar levels for individuals with insulin resistance	1,000 mg	1,000 mg

CHAPTER 10

BEAT HEART DISEASE

My son, do not forget my teaching, but let your heart keep my commandments; for length of days and long life and peace will they add to you.

—PROVERBS 3:1–2

HEART DISEASE IS a killer. Have you ever heard of someone dying of a heart attack who was the least likely person you would expect to suffer heart disease? Seemingly healthy people in their prime—including football stars and other athletes—fall over dead, sometimes even after just having passed a physical at their doctor's office. Contrary to what it might look like on the surface, the heart attack did not take place as suddenly as it seemed. More than likely, underlying problems had remained undetected and untreated in that person's body—perhaps for years—that eventually killed him or her.

You may be aware that the cardiovascular system is the system in your body that circulates blood, carrying life-giving oxygen *to* and poisonous waste products *from* your vital organs. The word *cardiovascular* means "pertaining to the heart and the blood vessels." Therefore, *cardiovascular disease* is any disease that would affect those areas of the body.

Cardiovascular disease is the number-one killer today—even among Christians—often striking suddenly and without warning. About one quarter of all deaths in America are due to heart disease, and it is the leading cause of death for Americans.[1] This crisis affects us all, whether we are facing it in our own bodies or watching it happen to someone we love. But the good news is that it is possible to prevent and even reverse cardiovascular disease before it becomes deadly.

Although our archenemy Satan, whose purpose is to kill, steal, and destroy (John 10:10), would like to wipe out as many people in the body of Christ as possible through heart or vascular illness, God has provided everything that our bodies need to counteract this deadly killer. Our first step is to educate ourselves about our bodies and how they function, and then learn the methods and substances that God would have us use to restore and maintain our body's health.

As you will see in this chapter, cardiovascular disease involves more than just heart attacks. It encompasses a host of ailments that affect the heart, blood vessels, veins, and arteries. We will examine the most common of these ailments, which may be affecting your health without your even being aware of them. How much do you know about your heart?

ANATOMY OF THE HEART

The human heart is a strong muscle used to pump blood through the arteries and veins, dispensing important nutrients and oxygen and carrying waste material away from the cells. There are four chambers in the heart. The two upper chambers—the atria—are smaller than the two lower chambers—the ventricles—the large pumping chambers that propel the blood out of the heart and throughout the body. The right ventricle pumps blood to the lungs, while the left ventricle pumps blood to the rest of the body.

Arrhythmia: irregular heartbeats

Most people who experience arrhythmia don't go in to see their doctor and say, "I've got an irregular heartbeat, Doc. I think I might have an arrhythmia." Many people aren't even aware that they are experiencing an arrhythmia. Their observations may be something like, "My heart has been doing flip-flops lately," or, "I've been having palpitations." Sometimes they may feel as if their heart has paused or skipped a beat, which can be quite frightening to people who don't understand what is happening to them. Some people may even begin to wonder if they are about to have a heart attack. If their heartbeat pauses for longer than a beat, they wonder if it will start to beat again!

Arrhythmia, or irregular heartbeat, is a very common condition. In fact, all of us have a type of irregular heartbeat called a *sinus arrhythmia*, which is actually quite normal. If you were to be sitting in your chair, resting and breathing at a normal pace, and you happened to take your pulse at that time, you might notice that your pulse was not occurring at an entirely steady rate. It may speed up slightly and then just slow back down. Heart rates often vary according to a person's breathing pattern or other changes that are occurring in the body. Becoming aware that this is a normal occurrence will keep you from feeling alarmed.

A study was done on a group of medical students during which each of them was hooked up to an electrocardiogram that measured their resting heart rates. Even though these were young, healthy, college-age students, every single one of them—that's *100 percent*—had irregularities in their heart rhythms. Most students were completely unaware of their arrhythmia, and almost all of the irregularities were benign.[2]

Sinus arrhythmia is nothing at all about which to be alarmed. In fact, it is a good idea for you to become aware of the usual heart rate patterns that occur in your own body so that you can detect the more dangerous forms of arrhythmia that could occur in case of disease.

Bradycardia

One heart irregularity to which we must pay much closer attention is *bradycardia*. The root word *brady* means "slow," and *cardia*, of course, refers to the heart; therefore, bradycardia indicates that a person's heart is beating more slowly than it should.

The immediate question that probably comes to your mind is, *How do I know how slow is too slow?* First of all, as I have stated, it is important for you to get to know your own body. Many athletes who are in peak physical condition will have slower heart rates than people who are not in shape. I am a runner, and because I run on a regular basis, my own heart rate is lower than that of many people. But on the average, if your resting heart rate drops to fifty beats per minute or lower, you could be experiencing bradycardia. If that is the case, you should get your heart rate checked by your doctor.

God placed within your heart a natural defense against bradycardia. A misfiring of the electrical impulses of the heart, which could cause bradycardia, is controlled by the *sinoatrial node*, a "natural pacemaker." When it triggers a conduction pathway, electricity passes through the A-V node (atrioventricular node) of the heart tissue, which in turn causes the lower ventricles of the heart to contract and pump blood. When everything is functioning normally, the sinus node fires regularly, usually around seventy to seventy-five beats per minute. But if there is a problem, perhaps some scar tissue or other disruption of the electrical impulse, the ventricles do not receive the signal to contract. At that point your heart would conceivably stop beating and you would be in serious trouble, except for God's wonderful protective design.

God designed your heart to keep beating even if there is a disruption of the electrical signals; the ventricles will contract on their own, continuing to send life-giving blood to your brain and other vital organs. It is a survival mechanism, designed to keep you alive. The problem is that the contractions will only occur at about forty beats per minute. At that rate, you will notice that something is very wrong. Because there isn't enough blood circulating, you will become light-headed, dizzy, perhaps even disoriented. When this happens, it is time to seek medical attention. Bradycardia—slow heartbeat—can signal that there is a problem with this built-in pacemaker that God designed. If it is not kicking in correctly, your heart rate can drop dangerously low, and your vital organs—especially the brain—can experience a devastating lack of blood flow.

What can be done to correct this potentially dangerous situation? First of all, as I mentioned earlier, accurate, specific knowledge about what is wrong is helpful to let you know how to target your prayers. You can begin to pray specifically for the sinus node, that it would function normally and that the nerve impulses it sends would flow correctly through the heart and cause it to pump blood in the way that it should. A medical answer for people whose built-in pacemakers are not functioning correctly sometimes involves inserting a surgically implanted pacemaker into the heart to keep it beating regularly.

There are more causes of bradycardia than the misfiring of the electrical impulses in the heart. An abnormally low heart rate can also be an indication of a thyroid problem. Because the thyroid gland is the master gland that controls metabolism in the body—including heart rate—if the hormones from the thyroid are not at the correct level, your heart rate can slow down. Your doctor can order a simple test called an *Ultrasensitive TSH* that will test your thyroid hormone levels to rule out this problem.

Tachycardia

At the opposite extreme from bradycardia is the condition of *tachycardia*, meaning a heart rate that is too rapid. The prefix *tachy* means "fast," and, again, *cardia* means "heart." Tachycardia is generally defined as a resting heart rate that is over one hundred beats per minute.

Tachycardia can be caused by a variety of conditions. One of the first things that doctors will check for is anemia, or a low blood count. Some people with anemia will experience heart rates of up to one hundred twenty beats per minute. If you have a drop in your hemoglobin, which carries oxygen to your tissues and organs, you will start to experience a lack of oxygen in those tissues. God has designed the body to signal the heart to beat faster when this occurs so that more blood will be carried throughout the body in a shorter period of time. We truly are fearfully and wonderfully made! If you are experiencing an unusually high heart rate, ask your doctor to perform a simple blood test (CBC) to determine whether or not you are anemic. It can tell you the levels of iron in your blood, the number of red blood cells, and so on; the CBC can also help point to a solution to your heart rate problem.

Tachycardia can also be a symptom of an underlying infection somewhere in the body. On the average, for every degree of above-normal temperature (fever) in the body, the heart rate goes up ten beats per minute. So if your heart begins to beat faster on a consistent basis, begin to ask God to show you if there are any infections lurking in your body of which you might be unaware. Have your doctor perform a check of your white blood cell count to see if your body is under attack. Perhaps your immune system has been weakened by poor nutrition or some other reason. A weakened immune system can be strengthened by increasing appropriate supplement support that will help your body fight off infection.

Paroxysmal supraventricular tachycardia

Another type of arrhythmia, called *paroxysmal supraventricular tachycardia (PSVT)*, can be as frightening as it sounds! Most arrhythmias cause you to feel as though your heart has just done a flip-flop or even skipped a beat or two; those are usually premature contractions of the atria, the upper chambers of the heart, and are generally benign. However, when PSVT occurs, you could be calmly sitting in an easy chair, breathing normally, when suddenly your heart takes off on a full-speed gallop, sometimes reaching a rate of 220 beats per minute. That's enough to get anyone's attention!

Many people who experience PSVT rush to the emergency room, convinced they are having a heart attack. However, what has happened is that the upper chambers of the heart begin to beat on their own at a super rate of speed. The lower chambers are not beating fast enough to keep up, so they begin to fill poorly with blood, causing you to feel nauseated, light-headed, or dizzy. Sometimes the problem lasts only a few seconds and then goes away, but it can last up to eight or ten hours, which is what usually causes a person to panic.

The enemy loves to plant fear in our hearts, and he is especially effective when he uses deceit to do so. The fact is that PSVT is usually a harmless phenomenon. Even in the emergency room one of the age-old treatments that doctors will use to treat it is one of the simplest: breathing into a paper bag. By doing so, the levels of carbon dioxide in your bloodstream are raised, which terminates the irregular heart rhythm. Some other tricks that are also effective include coughing as hard as possible, holding your breath for twenty seconds, or splashing cold water on your face. These simple treatments cause enough of a shock to your system that your heart rate is brought back to normal.

Isn't it amazing how something so frightening can be remedied by such simple methods? Many doctors' first response is to take out a prescription pad and give you a pill or two to take. But wouldn't a better approach to the problem be offering the patient a paper bag to breathe into, which could solve the problem simply? Paper bags don't have side effects! A good principle to follow is to try the simple solutions first before reaching for a pill or medication that could cause you further problems.

Atrial fibrillation

A more dangerous form of irregular heartbeat is called *atrial fibrillation*. The term *atrial* refers to the upper chambers of the heart, and *fibrillation* means "a shaking or a quivering motion." Therefore, atrial fibrillation is a quivering that occurs in the upper chambers of the heart. A good comparison to what goes on would be that of the agitator in the washing machine that slaps the clothes around in the water to get them clean. However, when the atria of the heart begin to agitate in this manner, they aren't stirring up soap and water; they're affecting platelets in the bloodstream. When these platelets are stimulated in such a manner, they begin to stick together, forming the dangerous condition of a blood clot. The blood clot then finds its way into the ventricles of the heart, where it can be pumped into the carotid or vertebral arteries, go straight to the brain, and cause a stroke.

Because atrial fibrillation can cause such a dangerous situation, it is important to have a checkup performed occasionally. Most people suffering from atrial fibrillation would not be able to feel it occurring in their chest. If the condition is diagnosed, there are several ways to treat it. The first course of action is to prevent the platelets in the blood from sticking together. For younger people (under the age of seventy), a simple dose of aspirin (325 milligrams per day) is effective. However, if a person is over the age of seventy, a blood thinner is usually required.

If you are using a blood thinner, you will need to have your blood monitored through tests to adjust the dosage. If your blood becomes too thin, you will have a tendency to bleed, but if it is not thin enough, it will not be effective in blocking the formation of blood clots in the heart. Interestingly if the blood clot tendency is prevented, even if the atrial fibrillation is not brought under control, the condition is usually no longer a health issue.

Sometimes atrial fibrillation can indicate a problem in one of the valves in the heart. I recommend that you ask your doctor to perform an echocardiogram to check for this condition. (He probably will anyway.) If a valve is too narrow or has developed stenosis (thickening), the blood may not be passing through it correctly and may be disrupting the beating of the heart.

If you are experiencing atrial fibrillation, arm yourself with the information you have just received and take it before the Lord in prayer. Begin to command your platelets, in the name of Jesus, to *not* clump themselves together or form blood clots in your heart. Speak to the atria of your heart and command them to beat regularly, in the manner that God intended. Seek the wisdom of the Father to know what pathway to take, whether it be a dose of aspirin or a regimen of blood thinners. Remember, He has a pathway to healing designed just for you.

Premature ventricular contraction

All of us will experience premature ventricular contractions (PVCs) at one time or another, but it is when they become a consistent pattern that they become very dangerous. In a normal heartbeat, just before the electrical impulse is fired, there is an instant of time called "repolarization." It occurs just after the completion of one heartbeat, when the heart is preparing to beat again. However, if the heart fires off too early, there will then be a long pause, and the ventricles of the heart will begin to overfill with blood. This causes the ventricles to stretch and then beat strongly to push all of the blood into the bloodstream. You will notice this strong heartbeat and will often have to pause for breath or cough in order to recover.

Many times premature ventricular contraction can be caused by stress, too much caffeine, or even stimulants found in over-the-counter cold medicines (pseudoephedrines). Most of the time the situation is benign. However, if there are three or more of this type of heartbeat that occur right in a row, something called *ventricular tachycardia*, or VT, occurs. When VT occurs, which involves several longer pauses in a row between heartbeats, there is no time for the heart to fill with blood. Suddenly there is a shortage of blood being pumped from the heart. People have been known to pass out at this point from the lack of circulation to their brains. Once this dangerous cycle has begun, the person may progress quickly from VT to a very serious problem called *ventricular fibrillation*.

You may be familiar with the term *ventricular fibrillation* from watching one of the many popular medical shows on television. When the doctor shouts out, "He's going into VFIB!" this is the condition to which he is referring. Ventricular fibrillation is very different from atrial fibrillation because it affects the large pumping chambers of the heart. If these chambers begin to quiver, they are not pumping blood effectively, and the person will die very quickly if drastic measures—usually an electrical shock to the heart—are not taken. I encourage you to seek medical advice if you are aware of a pattern of symptoms we described—feeling strong heartbeats that take your breath, especially if they occur continually.

NATURAL SUBSTANCES TO PREVENT OR REVERSE ARRHYTHMIA

God has provided several natural substances that have proven to be very effective in the prevention and treatment of these cardiovascular problems we have just discussed. As you seek to approach your situation in the simplest way first, I suggest you consider the following supplements as valid options, along with prayer and seeking medical advice.

Coenzyme Q_{10}
Coenzyme Q_{10} has proven effective in stabilizing abnormal rhythms of the heart, which is the primary cause of many forms of cardiovascular disease. A dosage of 50 milligrams per day will strengthen the heart muscle and allow it to beat with stability.

Magnesium
Right behind coenzyme Q_{10} in effectiveness against cardiovascular disease is magnesium. In fact, for years magnesium was used in hospital IVs to help stabilize patients' heart rates. Four hundred milligrams daily will stabilize the electrical disturbances in the heart.

Omega-3 fatty acids (fish oil)
There are many benefits to omega-3 oils, but one benefit that has been proven in medical journal studies is that omega-3 oils stabilize irregular heartbeats. You should take a dose of 2,000 milligrams per day.

Potassium
Potassium levels that are either too high or too low will frequently cause irregular heart rates. Generally a dose of 99 milligrams of potassium daily is sufficient.

Calcium

There are four basic forms of calcium, and I always tell my patients to get their calcium from more than one form. *Carbonate* (found in Tums), while the most common form of calcium, is not the most easily absorbed. *Citrate* is the most absorbable form, but *lactate* (found in milk) and *ascorbate* are also available. Calcium has a double benefit: it can both stabilize heart rate and lower blood pressure. You should take 500 milligrams of calcium per day.

It is best to combine these supplements in your regimen because their effect is synergistic, meaning their effectiveness multiplies when they are used together.

THE REAL CAUSES OF HEART ATTACKS

Two of the most frightening words that a person can hear are the words *heart attack*. That is understandable because of the history of tragedy heart attacks represent to lives and families. The good news is that new discoveries are making it possible for us to prevent heart attacks—and to do so in a natural way.

As I mentioned in the beginning of this chapter, it is often a mystery why seemingly healthy people—even athletes—can just keel over and die of a heart attack without any warning whatsoever. In fact, many people who have had heart attacks report having never had a symptom before their first heart attack occurred. The answer to this mystery lies in an understanding of how buildup of plaque in the arteries actually takes place.

For years doctors had believed that an artery was like a water pipe that slowly collected plaque over the years, causing a buildup that eventually blocked the artery and caused a heart attack. That is what I was taught in medical school, and it certainly seemed to be a logical explanation. Unfortunately, as we are just now starting to discover, it was wrong.

The arteries that are 90 percent blocked, we are learning, are *not* the arteries that cause most heart attacks! People with blocked arteries often experience *angina*, which is defined as chest pain on exertion. It is difficult for the blood to flow through their arteries when they exert themselves. But often in heart attacks, there is a sudden onset of chest pain, which begins in the middle of the chest and radiates outward, often through the left side and down the left arm.

What is happening is that fatty plaque develops not just within the artery itself but also in the *wall* of the artery. This plaque, which is covered by the lining of the arterial wall, builds up and actually causes the lining of the artery to rupture. When that happens, suddenly, the fatty material within the wall begins to protrude into the blood flow in the artery.

Because our bodies were created to repair themselves, when they detect any breach, such as the arterial rupture, the body's healing process signals a blood clot to form. In this case the effects of that natural healing process can be disastrous. Platelets begin to stick together, a clot begins to form, and in a period of a few minutes that clot fills up the artery, blocking blood flow. In addition, the artery itself begins to constrict in order to stop the flow of blood from the breach in the wall's lining—again, with disastrous consequences. The total effect results in myocardial infarction—heart attack.

HEART ATTACK PREVENTION

Fortunately, now that we are beginning to understand the true cause of most heart attacks, we are better equipped to prevent them. Preventive strategies such as lowering the LDL (bad) cholesterol, strengthening the arterial walls, preventing platelets from clotting, preventing hardening of the arteries, and removing saturated fat from your diet can go a long way toward lowering your risk of a heart attack.

God has made provision for our health—even for the prevention of heart attacks—and one of the keys to this provision, which I have mentioned, can be found in His Word. Consider its significance to the health of your heart:

> You must never eat any fat or blood.
> —LEVITICUS 3:17, NLT

> Then the LORD said to Moses, "Give the following instructions to the people of Israel. You must never eat fat, whether from cattle, sheep, or goats. The fat of an animal found dead or torn to pieces by wild animals must never be eaten, though it may be used for any other purpose. Anyone who eats fat from an animal presented as a special gift to the LORD will be cut off from the community. No matter where you live, you must never consume the blood of any bird or animal. Anyone who consumes blood will be cut off from the community."
> —LEVITICUS 7:22–27, NLT

The life of the body is in its blood.

—LEVITICUS 17:11, NLT

Have you ever noticed that many people have heart attacks shortly after they have finished consuming a huge meal that is often full of fatty foods? There is a much higher rate of heart attacks in people who have just consumed a meal that is high in saturated (animal) fats or trans-fatty acids from hydrogenated or partially hydrogenated oils. This fact is especially true among people who already have underlying coronary disease.[3]

The reason for this is that the fats contained in the food cause the coronary arteries to constrict and shut off the flow of blood in an already narrowed artery. Lack of blood flow to the heart then causes a myocardial infarction, otherwise known as a heart attack.

I find it interesting that God gave us instructions to keep us healthy in His written Word, which was written thousands of years ago. His command that we should never eat the fat or blood from an animal is now understood scientifically as a helpful prohibition to avoid the saturated fats found in meat—the fats known to be the most harmful to human beings. Other fats that God does not prohibit—fats found in certain vegetable oils, for example—have been found to be good for human consumption. The cultures that eat primarily these foods are remarkably healthier than those that consume primarily animal fat. Again, modern science proves that God knows what He is doing!

In His mercy God continues to provide natural ways of healing for those who violate His command regarding the consumption of animal fat. There are two substances that, when taken with a fatty meal, will help prevent the constriction of arteries: vitamin E and oatmeal. Eight hundred international units of vitamin E (D-alpha variety) can help stop the artery constriction that usually takes place after the consumption of a fatty meal. I generally recommend the vitamin E supplement because it is so much easier to take than eating a bowl of oatmeal after a steak dinner. I also recommend reducing your intake of these harmful fats, if not eliminating them altogether.

Hardening of the arteries

Hardening of the arteries is one of the leading causes of heart attacks and strokes. Scientists are finding that hardening of the arteries is really an inflammation in the arteries. Most of us think that hardening of the arteries is a condition in which solid calcium deposits form in the arteries just as calcium forms in the water pipes in our homes. This is not an accurate understanding of what is occurring.

The LDL (bad) cholesterol forms a solid or semisolid plaque or deposit that can stiffen artery walls. This plaque consists of white blood cells, smooth muscle cells, platelets, and other components, but it basically represents an inflammatory process in the plaque. There are at least four approaches you can take to help prevent this deadly problem from attacking your body.

Congestive heart failure

Congestive heart failure occurs when there has been so much damage to the heart muscle that it cannot pump fast enough to prevent a buildup of fluid in the lungs. Many people with congestive heart failure also have swelling or edema in their ankles. These patients usually reach a point where their lung capacity is so limited that they cannot lie flat in bed because when they do, it is difficult to breathe. They also become out of breath quickly with any level of exertion.

Long before doctors understood what congestive heart failure was, they knew that a certain family of plants—the rose family, which includes *hawthorn extract*—was helpful in strengthening the contractions of the heart. Today we are rediscovering the uses of this invaluable natural substance.

Controlled studies have been conducted that show the benefits of hawthorn extract in the reversal of congestive heart failure. It has a direct effect on the electrical impulses of the heart, shortening the refractory time between heartbeats and allowing the heart to pump more fluid more effectively.[4]

PREVENTION OF HEART DISEASE

The best way to stop heart attacks from occurring is to prevent heart disease from developing altogether. There are many new breakthrough discoveries from the natural plant kingdom that are causing great strides in the prevention of cardiovascular disease. Perhaps the most astounding of these is *policosanol*.

Policosanol

For years people have been harvesting sugarcane in order to create that sweet substance so many of us use inordinately and that is actually very harmful to our bodies. In the production of sugar from sugarcane an amazing by-product is created that until recently was considered simply a waste product. It is called *policosanol,* a waxy substance now determined to be a potent cholesterol-lowering and heart-protective agent. To prevent atherosclerosis, or hardening of the arteries, the LDL (bad) levels of cholesterol need to be under 100, and the HDL (good) levels of cholesterol should be well above 40. One study showed that policosanol lowered the LDL (bad) cholesterol levels in patients 20 percent in just six to twelve weeks, rivaling the prescription medications Zocor, Lipitor, and Pravachol—and *without the side effects of the prescription medications!* [5]

Many of these cholesterol medications cause the sudden onset of muscle aches and pains, which can progress into a breakdown of muscle tissue. They can also cause serious liver damage. Policosanol caused none of these side effects. (The only side effect noted was weight loss—and none of the subjects complained about that!) In addition, policosanol was shown to raise the levels of HDL (good) cholesterol by 15 percent. [6] The recommended daily dose for policosanol is 10 milligrams.

God so often chooses the foolish things of the world to confound the wise. Who would have thought that a waste product of sugarcane could have such unbelievable healing properties? When you compare the side effects and the cost of prescription drugs to the good results possible with a natural substance such as policosanol, it becomes clear that God is providing the healing for His people that He promised in His Word.

Natural treatments for homocysteine

One major new risk factor in the development of heart disease and hardening arteries is the presence of homocysteine levels in the blood, because they are so strongly associated with arterial blockage. In fact, many doctors consider high levels of homocysteine as great a risk factor for heart disease as smoking. However, once again God has provided some natural remedies that help to lower the homocysteine levels in the blood.

Anyone with high homocysteine levels should be on a regimen of B_6 and B_{12} vitamins as well as folic acid. Additionally the chemical compound *trimethylglycine*, also known as *betaine*, has been shown to work in conjunction with the B vitamins in lowering homocysteine levels. Betaine actually is a methyl donor that is found in sugar beets.

Take 75 milligrams of vitamin B_6 (or 85 milligrams if you have heart problems or a strong family history), 100 micrograms of vitamin B_{12}, 600 mcg of folic acid, and 250 milligrams of betaine per day.

L-arginine

L-arginine, which helps to stimulate the production of nitric oxide in the body, should be included in any supplement program to protect the arteries. Nitric oxide is a natural chemical that dilates, or expands, the blood vessels in the body, including the coronary arteries. It is a good way to help increase the blood flow in blocked arteries or prevent blockage by keeping them expanded. L-arginine is also good to take after a fatty meal. As I stated previously, saturated fats cause the blood vessels to constrict, but taking L-arginine can counteract this effect. L-arginine should be taken at a dose of 1,000 milligrams per day.

Tocotrienols

Tocotrienols are actually cousins of vitamin E; they can be found in rice and rice bran. When taken in conjunction with policosanol, tocotrienols work even better than vitamin E to lower cholesterol and prevent platelets from sticking to the walls of the arteries. A mixed tocotrienol complex should be taken at a dose of 100 milligrams per day.

Take low-dose aspirin

Amazingly half the people with these plaques that can clog the arteries have normal cholesterol levels. It is the initial damage to the artery lining caused by the bad cholesterol that sets the stage for inflammation. This is why one low-dose (81 milligrams) "enteric-coated" baby aspirin can work wonders in preventing heart disease—it stops the inflammation. (The term "enteric-coated" should appear on the label of the bottle.) Interestingly regular aspirin (325 milligrams) may not be as effective as the low-dose aspirin.

Take antioxidants

Why does cholesterol damage the arteries? Damage is caused by the oxidation or breakdown of the LDL cholesterol, which enables it to harm the healthy cells lining the arteries. This is why it is so critical to provide antioxidants in the form of vitamin E (800 international units daily), vitamin C (2,000 milligrams daily), and selenium (200 micrograms daily), along with others, such as the carotenes and coenzyme Q_{10}.

Garlic

Garlic is an effective cholesterol-lowering agent when used in combination with the other substances we have listed. Garlic bulb extract should be taken at a dose of 120 milligrams per day.

Green tea

Drinking one cup of green tea per day has an effect on blood vessel walls, making them more elastic and better able to expand to allow a free flow of blood. Obviously this can significantly lower a person's risk of developing heart disease or suffering a stroke.

ESSENTIAL NUTRIENTS FOR A HEALTHY HEART		
Nutrient	**Effect**	**Daily Dosage**
L-arginine	Amino acid important in blood vessel regulation and cardiac function	1,000 mg
Betaine	Nutrient that protects the heart by regulating homocysteine levels	250 mg
Coenzyme Q_{10}	Nutrient essential to energy production in the heart and muscles	50 mg
Garlic bulb extract	Herb with numerous phytochemicals that help normalize blood pressure, reduce platelet stickiness, and regulate blood lipid levels	120 mg
Green tea leaf extract	Natural source of catechin antioxidants that protect tissues from free-radical damage	150 mg
Magnesium	Mineral concentrated in heart tissue and needed for energy metabolism in the heart	400 mg
Policosanol	Plant derivative that supports healthy cholesterol levels	10 mg
Mixed tocotrienol complex	Part of the vitamin E complex with important antioxidant and cholesterol-regulating activity	100 mg
Vitamin B_6	Essential vitamin that protects the heart by lowering homocysteine levels	10 mg
Vitamin B_{12}	Essential vitamin that protects the heart by lowering homocysteine levels	100 mcg

ESSENTIAL NUTRIENTS FOR A HEALTHY HEART		
Nutrient	**Effect**	**Daily Dosage**
Potassium	Helps regulate heart rhythm	99 mg
Calcium	Stabilizes heart rate and lowers blood pressure	500 mg

CHAPTER 11

LOWER BLOOD PRESSURE—NATURALLY

He will redeem their life from oppression and violence;
and precious shall be their blood in His sight.
—PSALM 72:14, NKJV

HIGH BLOOD PRESSURE is accurately called the silent killer. It is often the root cause of many other health problems, especially heart disease. As blood pressure readings approach 140/90 and above, a silent but deadly process begins weakening the body. Strain is placed on the heart muscle, and thickening in the pumping chamber of the heart (left ventricular hypertrophy) occurs. The incidence of heart attack and stroke begins to increase, and the kidneys begin suffering damage.

Many people believe that if their blood pressure is up, they will have some visible sign such as headaches or nosebleeds—but these are the exception. Usually there is no warning of high blood pressure until something breaks. By then it is a major battle to overcome the problem.

Unfortunately even when high blood pressure—also known as *hypertension*—is caught in time, many of the medications used by medical doctors to lower it have detrimental side effects, are rather expensive even with health insurance, and can be dangerous when combined with other drugs or certain foods.

God has a better way! The Bible tells us that "the leaves of the tree were for the healing of the nations" (Rev. 22:2). There are three natural supplements that, when used on a daily basis, can lower blood pressure naturally *and with no side effects!*

POTASSIUM

There are many studies that indicate the power of potassium to reduce blood pressure. I have found potassium to effectively protect the kidneys also because of its role in protecting the lining of blood vessels from damage. Consuming five or more servings of fruits and vegetables daily is the ideal way to obtain sufficient potassium. I also recommend potassium in the citrate form at a total of 99 milligrams daily. Taking the supplement will ensure constant blood levels, and your dietary intake of fruits and vegetables can simply build on this consistent level.

POLYPHENOLS

Polyphenols are important compounds found in numerous foods. One particular association has been reported between certain polyphenols found in olive oil and the lowering of blood pressure.

A study reported in one medical journal noted that patients using 1 to 2 tablespoons of olive oil daily showed a marked reduction in the required dosage of blood pressure medications.[1] In fact, patients who were on antihypertensive medications were frequently able to cut their medicine dosage in half after only a few months.

In these studies a cold-pressed extra-virgin olive oil was utilized. Other oils, such as polyunsaturated oils, do not have these polyphenols present and do not produce a reduction in blood pressure. The compounds contained in the olive oil stimulate the production of a natural substance known as *nitric oxide*, already present in the human body.

Nitric oxide is important because it tends to relax and dilate blood vessels, which results in blood pressure reduction. These phenols also function as antioxidants that reduce the damaging effects of free-radical compounds that can affect blood vessels.

Amazingly almost one-fourth of the patients in this study who were using olive oil were able to control their blood pressure without any prescription drugs![2] It is interesting to note that olive oil is an important component of the Mediterranean Diet. This may be one of many reasons that countries around the Mediterranean region have some of the lowest recorded rates of heart disease in the world.

MAGNESIUM

Magnesium is an increasingly important mineral. Studies conducted at Harvard University that looked at health habits among health professionals found that those who consumed higher amounts of magnesium in the form of fruits and vegetables had significantly lower blood pressure.[3]

Another study, known as the Honolulu Heart Study, showed that magnesium was the most consistent substance that correlated with lowering the systolic and diastolic blood pressure. (Systolic blood pressure, the upper number, is the pressure that occurs when the heart beats; diastolic blood pressure, the lower number, measures the relaxation of the heart between beats.) This study consistently showed that the lower the blood magnesium levels, the higher the risk of heart attacks and the development of high blood pressure.[4]

Low magnesium levels also correlated with hardening of the arteries and the accumulation of cholesterol plaque in the carotid arteries, which supply blood to the brain. Increased magnesium intake causes blood vessels to dilate, which in turn results in reduced blood pressure.

The dietary intake of magnesium in the United States has decreased by slightly more than 50 percent. At the same time we are facing an epidemic of high blood pressure, with approximately 75 million Americans currently diagnosed with hypertension.[5]

Because of this epidemic the time has come for magnesium supplementation. In fact, studies have been done using magnesium as a daily supplement. These studies indicated that both the systolic and diastolic blood pressures fell significantly during the period of the supplemental intake.[6]

Magnesium can also help prevent heart palpitations and improve cholesterol levels. Even greater benefits are noted when the magnesium is taken with a potassium supplement and when salt is restricted in the diet.

YES, WE HAVE NO BANANAS!

It is incredible to think that such a popular fruit as the banana can actually function as a blood-pressure-lowering agent, but more and more studies are pointing in that direction. We have known for some time that potassium can lower blood pressure to some extent and that bananas are high in potassium. More startling, however, is the recent discovery that bananas contain a natural compound used in our most popular antihypertensive medications!

One of the most popular classes of antihypertensives (blood pressure medications) is known as ACE inhibitors or ACE blockers. These are prescribed by physicians and rank near the top of the list for treating patients with high blood pressure, patients who have had heart attacks, and patients with congestive heart failure.

This class of drugs has also shown a protective effect on the kidneys of patients suffering kidney problems from diabetes. In fact, this is one of the safest types of blood pressure medication you can take. It is available in a one-pill-a-day dose form, and the newer varieties of the ACE blockers have almost no side effects.

The latest studies indicate that bananas contain a natural ACE blocker and can lower blood pressure up to 10 percent in patients who consume two bananas daily.[7]

TAKE ACTION!

Because high blood pressure can creep up slowly on a person, giving no warning signs until it is too late, it is so important to be proactive in preventing potential serious problems before they strike. *Have your blood pressure checked regularly.* If your doctor sees readings in the 130/80 range, it is time to take action. You should lose weight, exercise, increase your consumption of fruit—especially bananas—and consider taking supplements that can lower blood pressure, including garlic capsules (the equivalent of one clove daily).

If your readings are found to be consistently over 140/90, you may need to be on a one-pill-a-day prescription drug such as one of the ACE drugs. Once you start taking a drug, this does not mean that you will be on it for life. When lifestyle changes are made, many patients can decrease and even go off their blood pressure medicine. However, this must be done with close monitoring under the care of a physician.

Chapter 12

FIND RELIEF FROM
GASTROINTESTINAL DISORDERS

*Worship the LORD your God, and his blessing will be
on your food and water. I will take away sickness
from among you, and none will miscarry or be
barren in your land. I will give you a full life span.*

—EXODUS 23:25–26, NIV

YOU ARE WHAT you eat. When you were growing up, did you ever
hear this statement? Perhaps your mother made this declaration as
she was trying to get you to finish the vegetables on your plate. But was
she right? To a certain degree, she was, but a more accurate way to put
it would be, "You are what you eat *and* what you are able to absorb."
You can eat all the lima beans and green peas in the world, but unless
your body can absorb the nutrients in these vegetables, they won't do
you any good!

Like many other diseases in our culture, gastrointestinal disorders are on the rise. From ailments as common as heartburn to more
serious problems such as ulcers, acid reflux disease, and irritable bowel
syndrome, your digestive system is under attack. In a manner similar
to the immune system the digestive system is your first line of defense
against harmful agents in the world around you. All the nutrients your
body takes in pass through the digestive system. It is therefore crucial
to maintain gastrointestinal health and protect your body from attack
in this area.

FOUR PROCESSES OF DIGESTION

When you consider the digestive system, you may sensibly conclude that
its primary function is to digest food. That is true to an extent, but the
digestive system does much more than that for the body. There are four
major processes of digestion that will be helpful to understand for protecting your health:

1. Your body must *digest* food. Obviously you must take in the food and begin to break it down into various tiny components that the body can use for energy.

2. Your body must *eliminate* waste. Not every molecule of food that you take in can be used by the body, so what is not helpful or good for you must be sorted out and then removed.

3. Your body must *absorb* nutrients. As I mentioned, you can eat all the food you can fit into your stomach, but if you cannot absorb the nutrition available in that food, you will literally starve to death.

4. Your body must *normalize* its balance of "good" bacteria in your intestines. Otherwise known as *flora*, these good bacteria must be present in the colon for your body to function properly.

All four processes must be operating successfully to prevent or treat gastrointestinal disorders.

THE IMPORTANCE OF ENZYMES

When you ingest food into your body, digestion begins almost immediately. *Digestion* essentially means the breakdown of food into a form that can be absorbed by the body, and it cannot take place except in the presence of *enzymes*. There are many types of enzymes in the body, but for our purposes, we will examine key enzymes that are crucial to maintain your digestive health: amylase enzymes, which break down carbohydrates; lipase enzymes, which break down fats; and proteolytic enzymes, which break down proteins.

Through the work of these three types of enzymes, the entire gamut of nutrients available in the four major food groups are available to us. Lactase, an amylase enzyme, is necessary to break down the lactose that is found in milk. Some people do not produce this enzyme and are therefore lactose intolerant, or unable to drink milk without experiencing discomfort such as gas or bloating. Cellulase is another important amylase enzyme; it breaks down various vegetables that we eat.

Although they are produced in smaller amounts in various parts of the digestive tract, these enzymes are primarily secreted by the *pancreas*. The more enzymes the pancreas has to produce, the more it can be subjected to stress and fatigue. Therefore, one of the first steps to take to ensure the health of the digestive system is to supplement these primary enzymes as a part of your daily diet. Two hundred milligrams each should be taken daily of amylase, cellulase, lactase, lipase, and the protease enzymes.

A deficiency in any of these enzymes can result in a host of uncomfortable digestive problems: gas, bloating, diarrhea, or constipation. Without the proper amounts of enzymes necessary for digestion to take place, particles of food will pass through the body undigested and create these difficulties. A more serious effect of an enzyme deficiency, however, is fatigue. If problems are occurring at the digestive stage of the process, the food that is eaten is not broken down to a stage where it is absorbable by the body; therefore, the cells do not receive the nutrition that they need. Energy sources are quickly depleted, and you feel tired all the time.

One unusual ailment that is in early stages of research is called the *leaky gut syndrome*. This occurs when the proteolytic enzymes (protein digestion) are either not present in sufficient quantities or they are not functioning correctly. Leaky gut syndrome is believed to take place when larger protein molecules that have missed being properly digested migrate to the "gut," or small intestine, and are absorbed there rather than earlier in the digestive tract as God intended. This absorption in an inappropriate area creates an immunological response from the body, and it could be a cause of such immune-related problems as allergies or arthritis.

KONJAC ROOT: DIGESTIVE HELPER

The body cannot use everything you eat, so the "leftovers" must be eliminated. You have no doubt heard that it is important to eat more fiber. That is because fiber helps in this elimination process. The fibers that are most helpful are water soluble; this means they are able to absorb the water from the waste product. The konjac root, common to Japan and widely used by the Japanese, may contribute significantly to their health, giving them the longest average life span of any people in the world.

From the konjac root an unusual water-soluble fiber called glucomannan is formulated. The most amazing aspect about glucomannan is the sheer amount of water it can absorb: *two hundred times* its own weight in water! That means that very small amounts of it can have a big effect in absorbing watery waste in our intestines. Another significant aspect of glucomannan is that it aids in the absorption of cholesterol, all the while creating a feeling of fullness in the stomach, as it soaks up water and expands. It contains no calories and suppresses the appetite because of its volume. For these reasons the konjac root is becoming important as a weight-loss supplement.

Another important function of glucomannan, as mentioned previously, is its ability to regulate blood sugar. Through its immediate absorption of water, it slows down the absorption of sugar into the bloodstream; it can therefore be essential in leveling out the spikes and drops in blood sugar that are so harmful, especially to diabetics.

Yet another benefit of the konjac root is that it counters constipation. Glucomannan, after soaking up so much water, contains a fairly large water volume. As it passes through the intestines, it mixes with the stool and actually acts as a stool softener to prevent hard stools and constipation.

Water-soluble fibers, such as pectin or oat bran, will perform most of these functions, but the difference with the konjac root is that a very *small amount of glucomannan produces very big results!* I recommend 400 milligrams of glucomannan daily. With other fibers, people have to drink large glasses of fiber solutions that taste terrible in order to get the benefits that the concentrated levels in the konjac root provide with just a tiny amount. And because the amount is so small, it can be put inside of a capsule that can be swallowed and dissolved in the stomach. That's good news for a lot of people!

DID YOU SAY "GOOD BACTERIA"?

While problems in enzyme production will affect the digestive functions of the body, other potential difficulties can occur when the balance between "good" and "bad" bacteria in the intestines is disrupted. It seems strange to some people that any sort of bacteria could be beneficial, but it is true. God created these good bacteria, or flora, to live in our intestines and overwhelm the bad bacteria that could cause infections or other serious illnesses. There are over four hundred different species of helpful flora naturally residing in the colon, two of the most common being *bifidobacterium* and *lactobacillus*.

One of the most interesting terms used to describe this type of bacteria is *probiotic*. When you consider the literal meaning of that word, it has special significance to us as Christians who understand that God created our bodies to be the temple, or dwelling place, for His Holy Spirit. *Probiotic* means "pro life" or "promoting life." When, for instance, you inadvertently drink polluted water that contains harmful bacteria, the probiotic bacteria in your digestive system go to work and attack the foreign invader, literally promoting life in your body.

Another function of the flora is to keep the normal yeast levels of the intestines in balance. If this gets out of hand, especially in women, commonly recurring yeast infections will take place. An underlying cause of these infections is an insufficient amount of good bacteria in the colon. Additionally some forms of bacteria in the intestines assist in the production of enzymes, one of which is lactase, the enzyme discussed earlier that breaks down the lactose sugars in milk and dairy products. One potential cause of lactose intolerance, then, could be a deficiency in the bacteria that produce lactase.

WHY ANTIBIOTICS CAN ACTUALLY BE HARMFUL

Again, the common misconception that most people have is that all bacteria are bad, and therefore all antibiotics must be good. But take into account our definition of the probiotic bacteria: If *probiotic* means "promote life," then what might *antibiotic* mean? Yes, antibiotics are literally "against life," most commonly against the life of bad bacteria, but when you ingest an antibiotic into your body, it doesn't know the difference between good bacteria and bad bacteria. It kills them all.

Sometimes a round of antibiotics is necessary to knock out a bacterial infection or a case of pneumonia, but I must emphasize that if you have taken antibiotics for whatever reason, you must recolonize your intestines with the good flora that were wiped out by the antibiotics.

The following substances may be taken to restore a normal balance of bacteria in the intestines:

+ Arabinogalactan, 250 milligrams per day
+ Fructooligosaccharides, 100 milligrams per day
+ Lactobacillus, 150 milligrams per day

You may be saying to yourself, "I haven't needed to take an antibiotic for years!" Even if that is the case, it is a good idea to recolonize your intestines periodically. You may not have been prescribed an antibiotic by your doctor, but have you eaten chicken lately? Poultry, among other animals raised for our food supply, are regularly treated with antibiotics, which remain in their system right up until the time we take that first bite. And every bite thereafter is slowly killing off the good bacteria in your colon.

For these reasons, it is important for all of us to supplement our digestive systems with probiotics, enzymes, and the fiber found in the konjac root. Begin to add these things to your diet, and watch God begin to restore your digestive health.

TREAT ACID REFLUX DISEASE NATURALLY

Now that I have discussed the basics of the digestive system, let's talk about some specific gastrointestinal disorders, beginning with acid reflux. Periodic episodes of heartburn caused by acid reflux are very common. However, when these episodes occur frequently, they can become much more than just a nuisance. In fact, frequent episodes of acid reflux (technically known as *gastroesophageal reflux disease*, or GERD) can increase the potential risk of esophageal cancer by causing changes in the cells lining the esophagus.

Here are five helpful suggestions that have been proven to quench heartburn without the use of prescription medicine. They are simple at-home techniques that I would recommend you try before seeking help from your doctor. However, if you are consistently experiencing more than three episodes of heartburn a week, you should see your doctor as soon as possible to help prevent developing scar tissue in your esophagus.

1. Eat large meals early and light meals later.

Many people skip breakfast, eat a small lunch, and consume their largest meal in the evening. This is just the opposite of the way people used to eat, and opposite of the way God designed our bodies to function. The change in our eating patterns combined with increased obesity has produced increasing problems with esophageal disease.

There is a muscular valve known as a *sphincter* between the esophagus and the stomach. The lining of the stomach is designed to handle a high acid level, but if this acid "refluxes," or backs up, into the esophagus, problems can occur. The cells lining the esophagus are not designed to handle high acid levels. The acid can cause severe damage and even erosions and inflammation in the esophagus that can produce the symptoms of heartburn.

When you eat late in the evening, large amounts of food are in the stomach when you lie down at night, producing pressure on the muscular sphincter. If you are carrying extra pounds, it produces additional pressure on the stomach, which in turn causes more acid to enter the esophagus. The simple habit of eating a light meal early in the evening can dramatically reduce the symptoms of reflux.

2. Raise the head of your bed.

By placing a small block of wood such as a two-by-four (or even a four-by-four-inch block, in some cases) under the head of the bed, you can elevate the entire bed. This prevents the return of acid into the esophagus and helps contain the acid in the stomach where it belongs. Adding an extra pillow or two under your head can actually make the problem worse because of the angle created between the esophagus and the stomach.

3. Avoid the three "bad guys": peppermint candy, coffee, and chocolate.

There are certain substances that can weaken the tone or strength of the sphincter muscle, allowing acid to reflux. These include coffee, peppermint candy, and chocolate. Isn't it ironic that many times after a meal at a restaurant, we have a cup of coffee, a peppermint candy, or a chocolate mint?

4. Drink more water.

A simple remedy for heartburn that has proven effective is to increase your daily consumption of water. The water tends to wash the acid off the wall of the esophagus.

5. Use antacids with caution.

If you need to use an occasional antacid, remember that the liquid antacids are better than the tablets because they tend to adhere to the esophagus, forming a protective coating. Over-the-counter medications known as H2 blockers can be used on occasion, but as we get older, the stomach tends to produce less acid, and the chronic use of these medications to neutralize acid can sometimes interfere with digestion.

NATURAL RELIEF FOR IRRITABLE BOWEL SYNDROME

This unpleasant syndrome affects millions of people. Irritable bowel syndrome (formerly known as spastic colon) can be a very frustrating and troublesome syndrome. This has been one of the most frustrating disorders facing the medical profession. In fact, it is the number-one referral made by family physicians to GI specialists (gastroenterologists).

Irritable bowel syndrome (IBS)—not to be confused with inflammatory bowel disease, such as ulcerative colitis or Crohn's disease—affects millions of people. The exact cause is still not fully understood, but it appears to be a problem with the transmission of nerve impulses affecting the nerve endings to the smooth muscles in the GI tract.

We also know that it has been associated with periods of high stress. Symptoms include abdominal bloating and cramping, excessive gas, and either diarrhea or constipation or alternating between the two.

Peppermint oil

An effective natural treatment for irritable bowel syndrome is enteric-coated peppermint oil. Research has indicated that the oil found in the peppermint plant can relax smooth muscles in the colon. Prescription muscle relaxants (known as *antispasmodics*) can cause numerous side effects, but the peppermint oil found in the plant kingdom has no side effects.[1] Peppermint oil has been found by several studies throughout the years to ease the symptoms of irritable bowel syndrome.[2]

There is one small problem with peppermint oil, however. In the last chapter we listed peppermint as a major irritant of acid reflux. If you have acid reflux disease as well as irritable bowel syndrome, it is imperative that you take the coated capsule form of the peppermint oil so that the oil will be absorbed in the intestine rather than in the stomach.

Researchers in Britain have recorded a nearly 50 percent reduction in colon spasms after peppermint oil was introduced into the colon. The capsules are available in a standardized, coated form that contains 0.2 milliliters of peppermint oil. One to two capsules daily between meals were used in the study.[3]

Other treatments for irritable bowel syndrome

Believe me, if you are suffering from severe symptoms of irritable bowel syndrome, you want *relief*. Sometimes a safe prescription medication may be required to relax the smooth muscle. Smooth muscle relaxants that have been proven effective include dicyclomine, mebeverine, and trimebutine. Amitiza and Linzess are prescriptions that can be used to treat IBS with constipation. Lotronex and Xifaxan can treat IBS with diarrhea. At least thirteen out of sixteen studies showed an improvement in symptoms while patients were on these medications.[4]

Other traditional treatments for irritable bowel syndrome include psyllium and wheat bran, although these are not as effective and can cause gas in quite a few patients. If peppermint oil capsules do not relieve the symptoms, try adding very small amounts of wheat bran. (An ideal amount would be ¼ cup of Kellogg's Bran Buds cereal.)

ESSENTIAL NUTRIENTS TO KEEP YOUR SYSTEM ON TRACK		
Nutrient	**Effect**	**Daily Dosage**
Amylase	Enzyme that helps in the digestion of carbohydrates	200 mg
Cellulase	Enzyme that helps in the digestion of cellulose, a fiber found in many fruits and vegetables	200 mg
Lactase	Enzyme that improves the digestion of lactose (milk sugar)	200 mg
Lipase	Enzyme that helps in the digestion of fats	200 mg
Protease I	Enzyme that helps in the digestion of meat proteins and helps reduce inflammation	200 mg
Protease II	Enzyme that helps in the digestion of plant proteins and helps reduce inflammation	200 mg
Protease III	Enzyme that helps in the digestion of milk proteins and helps reduce inflammation	200 mg
Glucomannan	Natural source of soluble fiber that helps eliminate toxins, enhance healthy blood sugar levels, reduce bloating, improve stool transit time and stool weight, support healthy cholesterol and fat metabolism, and create bulk for healthy regularity and elimination	400 mg
Arabinogalactan	Fiber-like substance that promotes the growth of friendly bacteria in the gut while suppressing the growth of harmful organisms	250 mg
Fructooligo-saccharides	Fiber-like substance that helps reduce bad bacteria while supporting friendly bacteria	100 mg

ESSENTIAL NUTRIENTS TO KEEP YOUR SYSTEM ON TRACK		
Nutrient	**Effect**	**Daily Dosage**
Lactobacillus sporogenes	Beneficial intestinal organism that reduces population of harmful organisms	150 mg

CHAPTER 13

PROTECT YOURSELF FROM COLDS AND FLU

*I will not afflict you with any of the diseases
with which I have afflicted the Egyptians.
For I am the LORD who heals you.*

—EXODUS 15:26

EVERYBODY HAS HAD it at least a few times. And when you see the clerk at the grocery store sneezing and coughing as she scans your merchandise, you realize that it could be coming your way soon.

Perhaps the most common ailments in the world are colds and flu viruses. We generally consider them just a nuisance to be endured, especially at certain times of the year. But if there were a way to prevent this misery and avoid the irritation and the loss of days of being productive in God's kingdom, wouldn't it be worth pursuing? For years scientists have been working on the elusive "cure" for the common cold, which they have yet to discover. Fortunately there are several natural ways to *prevent* it and to help protect yourself from ever catching a cold or coming down with the flu in the first place.

COLD OR FLU? SYMPTOMS AND TREATMENT

Because different viruses are involved in colds and the flu, it is helpful to recognize symptomatically which you are suffering. The following chart lists some of the common symptoms of each condition along with their intensity to help you differentiate between these common conditions.

Symptoms	Colds	Flu
Fever	Rare	Typical; high (102°–104° F); lasts three to four days
Headache	Rare	Prominent
General aches and pains	Light	Usual; often severe

Symptoms	Colds	Flu
Fatigue, weakness	Mild	Can last up to two to three weeks
Extreme exhaustion	Never	Early and prominent
Stuffy nose	Common	Sometimes
Sneezing	Usual	Sometimes
Sore throat	Common	Sometimes
Chest discomfort	Mild to moderate	Common; can become severe

Echinacea

Echinacea is familiar to many people as a popular immune-boosting herb. It ranks near the top of the list when it comes to countering colds or the flu. This herb not only prevents viral infections but also can fight them if they try to attack the body. Many of the patients that I see in my practice take echinacea during the cold and flu season simply as a preventive measure.

Echinacea works by stimulating the immune system, but it should not be taken on a daily basis for an extended period of time because tolerance can develop and cause it not to work as effectively. Echinacea should be used for four to eight weeks and then discontinued for at least two weeks. The recommended dosage is 2 to 3 teaspoons of the tincture daily, or you can take the standard-dose capsules and follow the directions on the label.

Garlic

Another important herb to use during the cold and flu season is garlic, which can fight viruses as well as bacteria. It is also effective for reducing the duration of colds and the flu. Again, garlic works by stimulating the immune system function. I recommend taking the capsule form daily, checking the label to be certain a capsule is the equivalent of one clove of fresh garlic.

Lesser-known herbs

There are several lesser-known herbs that are helpful for colds and the flu. For example, *thyme* has antiviral as well as antibacterial properties and can be made into a tea or taken as syrup. Another herb available at health food stores, known as *elder*, is a decongestant and an antiinflammatory that has traditionally been taken in the form of a hot tea.

Lemon balm is a helpful herb for easing headaches and the aching associated with flu symptoms.

Be certain also that you are on a good supplement program with a multivitamin and mineral supplement that includes B complex, zinc, and vitamin E, as well as chromium and selenium. All of these nutrients support immune system function. Remember the old chicken soup recipe? If you come down with symptoms, it can help to clear out mucus.

The body often develops a fever during a bout with the flu. Fevers stimulate the body's immune system and help it overcome the virus and bacterial infection. Of course, a fever that is too high can be dangerous, as we know. Be sure to force fluids, particularly if you have developed a fever. It is very important to do all you can to strengthen your body's defenses against these viral infections.

If you do come down with the flu despite all your best natural efforts, there are now prescription treatments available. Tamiflu, 75 milligrams twice daily, prescribed by your doctor, can dramatically decrease the flu symptoms if taken within the first two days of symptom onset.

NATURAL SINUS TREATMENTS

If you are always tired, constantly experience postnasal drainage, or feel that you have a cold all of the time, you could be afflicted with *chronic sinusitis*. It is important to distinguish an acute episode of sinusitis (inflammation of the sinus cavities) from chronic, persistent sinusitis.

Acute sinus problems begin with head congestion, thick green/yellow nasal drainage, postnasal mucus drainage, and extreme fatigue. These cold symptoms can last two or more weeks. *Chronic sinus* problems are identified by a low-grade infection, with periodic episodes of acute sinusitis. Patients often feel "sick all the time." They can have episodes of acute sinusitis, with the abovementioned symptoms, and three or more infections within six months, feeling good between episodes.

A third category of sinus problems involves *chronic inflammation* of the mucous membranes of the nose and sinus area but few, if any, infections. Doctors often mistakenly treat chronic sinusitis patients with antibiotics on a regular basis. This overuse of antibiotics can only lead to antibiotic-resistant "bugs," and eventually even the most powerful antibiotics will prove ineffective.

In patients who have persistent low-grade infection with periodic flare-ups of acute sinus problems and a feeling of being sick most of the time, antibiotics can be a real mistake, as they promote more infection and do not offer a cure. Overuse of antibiotics can actually contribute to the inflammation that aggravates the condition.

Chronic sinusitis is, by definition, an inflammation of the lining of the sinus cavities. These cavities occur over the eyes, beside the nose, and in other areas of the body. Air pollution and overuse of antibiotics can cause inflammation, infection, and even yeast overgrowth in these areas. The causes of the inflammation include stress, dry air, environmental or food allergies, and dental problems. These areas should all be addressed, and then the mucous membranes must be allowed to heal and the immune system function strengthened. Humidifiers, saline nasal sprays (non-medicated), and warm mists are helpful in soothing the mucous membrane lining. With central heating and air-conditioning systems, humidity plunges extremely low, drying out the mucous membranes and making them more vulnerable to inflammation and infection. Increasing daily water intake to 64 ounces is recommended.

Natural treatments

To stop the immediate problem of sinus inflammation, use steam and saline irrigation and brief courses of echinacea (three weeks on, one week off). Garlic should also be used daily (equivalent to one clove). I recommend 3,000–5,000 milligrams of vitamin C daily as well.

If these natural methods do not prove to be effective, I often recommend a minimally absorbable nasal anti-inflammatory spray such as Flonase for a short period of time, which can work wonders in many patients.

Many so-called sinus problems are really allergy problems. Secretions that build up in the sinus cavities and are not draining effectively usually cause true sinus problems (sinusitis), and these secretions can get infected.

There are some natural treatments and preventives that should be considered if excess mucus production, swelling, and other chronic respiratory problems are present. Since most of these problems are due to allergies, it is important to understand that allergies are caused by an *overactive* immune system that stimulates enzymes. These enzymes in turn release histamine and other chemicals that cause the symptoms.

There are four natural substances that block the enzymes causing the symptoms that I suggest you try if you are battling this problem: carotenoids, fish oil, quercetin, and resveratrol. Consider the brief explanation of each to help you decide how to use these helpful natural healers.

- Carotenoids: Typically found in yellow and orange foods, carotenoids should be increased not only in your diet but also in supplement form. They are cousins to beta-carotene and include alpha-carotene, lycopene, lutein, and other mixed carotenoids. A daily supplement containing 2.5 milligrams of these various carotenoids is recommended.

- Fish oil: By now you should be familiar with the essential nutrients containing the omega-3 fatty acids found in many types of fish. A total of 600 milligrams should be consumed daily.

- Quercetin: Flavonoids are another type of potent antioxidant. Quercetin is a flavonoid that is particularly helpful for allergy/sinus problems. A daily dosage of 25 milligrams is recommended.

- Resveratrol: Found in the skin of red grapes, resveratrol is also an anti-inflammatory agent that can help relieve allergy or sinus symptoms.

Other helpful tips

Dairy products should be avoided since they can cause inflammation and excess mucus production in some patients. Also avoid heavy exercise, which can weaken the immune system. Mild to moderate aerobic-type exercise is beneficial, however.

CHAPTER 14

TREAT HEADACHES AND DIZZINESS

Bless the Lord, O my soul, and all that is within
me, bless His holy name. Bless the Lord, O my
soul, and forget not all His benefits, who forgives
all your iniquities, who heals all your diseases.

—PSALM 103:1–3

HEADACHES AND DIZZINESS are among the most common ailments. Fortunately God is in the healing business, and He has provided natural treatments within His world to bring relief from these debilitating problems. Headaches are classified according to symptoms and cause. The vast majority of headaches can be relieved with simple relaxation techniques and by avoiding any unusual stimulation. Avoiding light and noise, relaxing in a quiet environment, and even praying can often relieve the pain of headaches.

TYPES OF HEADACHES

Categories of headaches range from simple stress or tension headaches to more severe problems such as brain tumors or temporal arteritis, which can be serious. The simple headache consists of a buzzing or pulsing discomfort in the head, and it can be related to high blood pressure, fever, stress, weather, or other causes. The following list may help you identify the type of headache(s) you experience.

Ice pick headaches
These are brief, stabbing headaches, which, although potentially frightening to many patients, are benign.

Tension headaches
This very common headache usually begins in the back of the head or neck area, or in the forehead or temple region, and spreads throughout the head. Frequently tension headaches occur on both sides of the head.

Cluster headaches

This type of headache is characterized by a piercing or burning pain, often occurring on one side of the head, usually in exactly the same place from one episode to another. These headaches occur on a regular basis for days or weeks at a time and then may disappear.

Migraine headaches

Migraine headaches are often referred to as "sick" headaches because vomiting, nausea, and vision problems often accompany them. These headaches are due to constrictions and dilations in blood vessels in the brain. Migraines are sometimes very difficult to diagnose as they may present only with blurred vision or partial loss of a vision field on one side.

Ocular migraine headache

This type of headache can cause a loss of peripheral vision. It is often hereditary.

Combination headache

The combination headache presents as a migraine headache followed by a dull, continuing pain afterward.

NATURAL PAIN RELIEF

Herbal treatments have been utilized to treat headaches. The natural, nonaddictive tranquilizer kava kava can help to relieve tension headaches. A migraine headache, however, which is caused by the expansion and constriction of blood vessels, is better treated with feverfew and ginkgo biloba. (Simply follow the instructions on the bottle for the appropriate dosage.)

Another treatment for headaches is to add just a few drops (four to five) of fresh lemon to a cup of black coffee and then sip it slowly. Caffeine is a well-known plant-derived substance that can help alleviate headaches by dilating the blood vessels in the brain. Another herbal treatment is to apply cold compresses that have had two to three drops of peppermint oil added to the cloth. Placing this against the painful area for fifteen minutes can relieve simple tension headaches.

A tried-and-true remedy used by many people is to make a compress of grated horseradish added to a small amount of water and applied to a cloth. The cloth is then applied to the neck area for up to five minutes. This compress can help to extinguish the tension type of headache pain.

Try not to get into the habit of using large amounts of

caffeine-containing over-the-counter compounds on a regular basis. This can lead to the phenomenon known as "rebound headaches." This simply means that as the caffeine levels decrease in your bloodstream, the headache will return, and you will require more and more caffeine-containing medication to stop it. If all other methods fail, there are some prescription medications available, such as Maxalt and Zomig, which may provide relief.

DIZZINESS

Dizziness is one of the most common neurological symptoms encountered in the medical practice. It is, in fact, second only to fatigue among "non-pain" symptoms. On one end of the scale dizziness is often a vague complaint that can be very brief and benign. By the same token it can extend to more serious diseases such as tumors or decreased blood flow to the brain.

The most common form of dizziness is known as *vertigo*. This term describes a sensation of motion when there is no motion or an exaggerated sense of motion in response to certain body movements. Vertigo may be a "spinning sensation," but it can also be a sense of falling forward, falling backward, or tumbling. Most forms of vertigo are related to inner ear problems and are often accompanied by nausea, vomiting, and occasional hearing loss.

The inner ear serves as a primary balance mechanism that involves canals lined with small hairlike structures. Within the canals are tiny crystals made of calcium carbonate, which press against the small hairs. These small crystals, known as *otoliths*, move as our body position changes, and gravity causes the crystals to press against hairs in different positions and send signals to the brain that orient us and keep us steady.

To maintain our balance, God created a complex series of organs that interact with each other. These include the inner ear, muscles, eyes, and even pressure receptors in the skin. All these organs provide input to the brain. The brain processes these signals to keep us in a steady balance.

Poor circulation to the brain can cause dizziness, as can certain viral or bacterial infections. Abnormally high or low blood pressure and brain tumors are also causes of dizziness. Anemia can result in dizziness as well, due to an inadequate oxygen supply to various organs.

Many patients become unnecessarily distraught due to a sudden onset of vertigo in the form of spinning or dizziness. However, although it can be extremely upsetting, in most cases it is benign and can be treated with simple measures. In fact, one of the most common forms of vertigo is called "benign positional vertigo." This is a spinning sensation that is associated with changes in head position, particularly when the person is lying down and suddenly sits up or stands. This form of vertigo tends to be brief and episodic, whereas viral or bacterial infections can cause an almost constant vertigo for several days that then disappears as the body's immune system functions take over.

When we suddenly rise from a sitting or stooped-over position and feel dizzy for a few seconds, it is caused by a temporary drop in blood pressure, known as *orthostatic hypotension*. If this occurs, it is almost always harmless, unless it occurs frequently—if that is the case, it could be indicating that the person has consistently low blood pressure.

To be certain there is not a more serious problem, a physician should evaluate any kind of persistent vertigo or dizziness. Occasionally an MRI is ordered to rule out any more dangerous conditions.

NATURAL RELIEF FROM DIZZINESS

God has provided several natural nutrients that can bring relief from the common problem of dizziness.

B vitamins

All of the B vitamins are important for normal brain and nervous system function. Taking a complex of the water-soluble B vitamins as part of your daily nutrient supplements is critical in maintaining a healthy nervous system. One hundred milligrams of vitamin B_3 taken three times daily can be very useful because of its effect on cerebral circulation. However, this dosage should not be taken if you have high blood pressure or liver problems.

Extra B complex, 100 milligrams two to three times daily, as well as extra B_6, 50 milligrams daily, may be helpful during periods of dizziness. Up to 1,000 micrograms of vitamin B_{12} daily can also be useful.

Other supplements

I recommend vitamin C, 2,000 milligrams daily, and vitamin E, 800 IU (natural form) daily, for dizziness. Coenzyme Q_{10}, when taken at a dose of 90 to 150 milligrams daily, can be useful during periods of dizziness as well.

Ginger

Certain herbs, such as powdered whole gingerroot in doses of 500 to 1,000 milligrams, can relieve dizziness and nausea. Ginger has been consumed for thousands of years to help treat dizziness. In one study of sailors who consumed 1 gram of powdered ginger two to three times daily, there were markedly reduced symptoms associated with seasickness such as vomiting and dizziness.[1] Ginger is available in capsules and can be taken thirty minutes before dizziness is anticipated and then every one to two hours thereafter.

Ginkgo

Ginkgo extract has been used for the treatment of vertigo in European countries. A typical dose should be 40 milligrams three times daily. Ginkgo extract can also improve blood circulation to the brain, as we have discussed.

Remember God's promise! If you diligently hearken to His voice, He will allow none of the diseases that affect the rest of the world to afflict you. (See Exodus 15:26.) As you develop an understanding of how headaches and dizziness attack your body, you will be better able to pray effectively and stand against them.

If you are experiencing a problem with headaches, sudden vertigo, or dizziness, you should pray about your specific pathway to healing. Let the Holy Spirit guide you and give you wisdom. Consider utilizing these natural treatments from God's plant kingdom. His desire is that you experience perfect health in your body and freedom from pain and dizzy spells.

CHAPTER 15

REMEDY VISION PROBLEMS

Moses was 120 years old when he died, yet his eyesight was perfect and he was as strong as a young man.
—DEUTERONOMY 34:7, TLB

W E NEVER LOSE our wonder of *enjoying the view!* Of all the senses in the human body, people cherish their vision more than any other. God understands this, and He has much to say in His Word about our eyesight. The writer of Proverbs instructs us clearly in this regard:

> Listen, son of mine, to what I say. Listen carefully. Keep these thoughts ever in mind; let them penetrate deep within your heart, for they will mean real life for you and radiant health....Look straight ahead; don't even turn your head to look. Watch your step. Stick to the path and be safe.
> —PROVERBS 4:20–22, 25–26, TLB

First of all, we are to pay attention to God's Word in order to receive the life and radiant health that God wants us to experience. But to do that, we are to look straight ahead of us to follow the path that He wants us to take. We need our eyesight to see His path! We especially need it to be able to study His Word, to keep it before our eyes so that the path remains clear.

The biblical record of Moses's death tells us something unusual about his health. It records for us the fact that Moses was one hundred twenty years old when he died and that his "eye was not dim, nor was his vitality diminished" (Deut. 34:7). The Living Bible paraphrase of this verse says, "His eyesight was perfect and he was as strong as a young man." Even in old age Moses did not experience cataracts, macular degeneration, or other vision problems that most of us experience as we get older. Thank God that we don't have to be like everybody else! He has a better way for His children.

Where should you turn when you begin to experience problems with your vision, those early symptoms that indicate something is going wrong, or worse, a full-blown diagnosis that could indicate encroaching blindness? Psalm 121 gives us the answer:

> I will lift up my eyes to the hills, from where does my help come?
> My help comes from the LORD, who made heaven and earth.
> —PSALM 121:1–2

God is our source of healing, and He is interested in curing both our spiritual and our physical blindness. He Himself is light, and He longs to dispel all darkness from our lives. Begin to seek Him for the pathway He would have you take to protect your precious eyesight. If you are already experiencing vision problems, ask Him to show you the pathway to healing He has prepared for you.

COMMON VISION PROBLEMS

Do you wear glasses or have eye problems? Are you concerned your vision isn't as sharp as it used to be? Your eyes are a delicate and sensitive part of your body, and aging, pollution, and sun exposure can weaken or damage them.

The primary vision problems that people have as they age include cataracts, macular degeneration, glaucoma, and retinopathy—the damage caused to the blood vessels of the eyes that is often related to diabetes. Let's take a look at each of these—what is occurring within the eye and the natural substances God has placed in our world that can stop or even reverse the process of these diseases.

Cataracts

Worldwide, the greatest cause of blindness is cataracts. In the United States there are surgical procedures that can stop blindness before it occurs, but when you consider that other countries don't have our technology, it's easy to see how cataracts can become such a problem.

Still, even here, when the doctor gives someone a diagnosis of cataracts, he generally sends the patient home "to see what develops." Well, usually what happens is the cataract gets worse until surgery becomes required to save the person's vision. Thousands of cataract surgeries are performed every year in this country—in fact, it is one of the most performed surgeries in the United States, right up there with appendectomies and gallbladder surgery.[1] About $6.8 billion is spent on cataract surgery every year in this country.[2] Wouldn't it be so much better to find a simpler way to stop the progression of cataracts at the very beginning stages?

Early signs that you are developing cataracts is that you begin to notice fogginess in your vision, a film over your eyes. Often while driving at night, the streetlights will begin to bother you because the way the light hits the cataract causes you to see what looks like halos around the lights. What is occurring is a degradation of the proteins within the lens of the eye, which causes a distortion in the person's vision.

Someone has said that if you live long enough, you are certain to develop cataracts. We as Christians don't accept that as truth because God has provided us with ways to counter the progressive damage to the eyes that occurs as we grow older.

Macular degeneration

Many older Americans, especially as they continue to age, have age-related macular degeneration. As one of the leading causes of irreversible blindness in the United States—not worldwide as we discussed with the problem of cataracts—we must ask what causes this problem, and more importantly, what can be done about it.

The *macula* is a small area in the back of the eye, in the retina where the central focus of light takes place. When eye doctors observe the macula in the retina, it appears as a small, concentrated yellow spot. Light passes into the eye through the lens and is magnified and focused down onto the retina, more specifically onto the macula where the sharpest focus of vision takes place.

Sunlight can be very harmful to the little macula. Within the prism of sunlight, the most dangerous rays are blue in color. If too many blue rays are allowed to come into contact with the macula, it destroys the nerve endings, and the person's vision will eventually begin to break down, causing *macular degeneration*.

Because macular degeneration can creep up on a person very slowly, it is important to pay attention to any early warning signs that may develop. One of the first symptoms is the loss of the central vision. A person begins to have trouble reading, doing close-up work, driving, seeing colors, or even distinguishing faces. The big tip-off is that people with macular degeneration can see things on the side of their vision much more clearly than right in the center. One of the first things people notice is that when they walk through a doorway, and they are trying to focus on the center of the door, the frames begin to seem wavy as they walk through the door—this is a classic early sign of macular degeneration.

There are two types of macular degeneration, wet and dry. Unfortunately, most individuals with the disease have dry macular degeneration, and there is no proven prescription that can help those individuals. The vast majority of the cases diagnosed by medical doctors are untreatable by the world's standards. Thank God that He is concerned about our eyesight, enough so that He has already put the necessary plants and natural substances in place to bring His light back into our eyes. As we will see, it is possible to completely halt the progression of macular degeneration by following God's dietary plan.

Diabetic retinopathy

As we discussed in the chapter on diabetes, this disease wreaks havoc on various areas of the body because of the negative effect it has on blood vessels that support so many different body organs. Diabetics are at a much greater risk of going blind than the general population because of the damage diabetes causes to the blood vessels of the retina.

Glaucoma

Glaucoma is a problem that occurs as pressure, for various reasons, increases in the eye. It is a relatively common cause of blindness, as the pressure in the eye exerts pressure on the optic nerve. Again, there is not much medical doctors can do to treat this condition, except to prescribe eye drops to try to lower the pressure and prevent blindness from taking place. The good news is that God has provided natural substances within His world that can make a greater difference, with less cost and fewer side effects to endure than conventional medications!

NATURAL REMEDIES FOR VISION PROBLEMS

Many of the natural substances help more than one type of vision problem. We will discuss the following substances that God has provided for us to maintain our good vision and correct any eye diseases or vision problems that might develop.

Lutein and zeaxanthin

The plant products *lutein* and *zeaxanthin* (types of yellow pigmentation) are found in various types of greens such as kale, collard greens, and spinach, and to a lesser degree in romaine lettuce, broccoli, zucchini, squash, green peas, brussels sprouts, and sweet corn.

These substances work to help prevent or stop the progress of macular degeneration by enhancing the yellow pigmentation of the macula, the pigmentation that is lost upon exposure to the sunlight. It literally functions as a sunscreen, blocking these most dangerous rays, the blue rays of the prism. Unfortunately, as our diets have worsened throughout the last several decades, most Americans do not consume enough kale and spinach to support the lutein levels that are needed to maintain good eyesight. Our poor diets have had a direct effect on the number of cases of macular degeneration that are now being reported. This is an example of how many people who, because they have ignored God's dietary laws, have made themselves vulnerable to a common cause of irreversible blindness.

But let's consider how easy it is to prevent. Every time you eat a big plate of spinach, you are literally putting a pair of heavy-duty sunglasses on the back of your eyes and protecting your eyesight from any potential damage from the sun! Fortunately, since the thought of kale and spinach doesn't appeal to many of us, you can also take lutein and zeaxanthin in supplement form. I recommend 6 milligrams per day.

These two nutrients are very helpful in preventing macular degeneration among most people, but it is especially important for those people who have the greatest risk of developing the disease. These people would include those who work or spend a great deal of time outside, being exposed to the sun's rays, or those who have blue or light-colored eyes, which are not able to filter out the harmful rays of the sun. If you have already been diagnosed with macular degeneration, take heart. Studies have shown that the pigments that have been lost can actually be restored through supplementation with lutein and zeaxanthin. In fact, within forty days of beginning a lutein supplement, studies have shown up to a 40 percent increase in the amount of protective yellow pigment present in the macula.[3]

Bilberry

In World War II, Royal Air Force pilots from Great Britain began noticing that when they ate bilberry jam and toast just before a night flight, there was a significant improvement in their night vision as they flew their fighter planes over enemy territory. The curiosity of scientists was aroused, and they began experiments to see if bilberry jam actually improved eyesight. In fact, they discovered that bilberry—a cousin of the blueberry—causes significant improvement in patients with macular degeneration.

Bilberry is also helpful for retinopathy, the damage done by diabetes to the retinal blood vessels, as well as for cataracts. When most doctors diagnose cataracts, they generally send the patient home until the problem escalates to the point where surgery is necessary. But if, at that time, the patient begins a regimen of bilberry, the progression of the cataract can be halted in its tracks. A dose of 40 milligrams per day is sufficient.

Eyebright

Eyebright comes from the Euphrasia plant, which grows wild throughout Europe. For centuries it has been used on that continent to relieve minor eye problems, especially those that deal with irritation, such as watery eyes caused by allergies, hay fever, or conjunctivitis. Although eyebright does not actually counter some of the more major diseases of the eye, it does help to alleviate some of the worst symptoms associated with these diseases. I recommend 10 milligrams of eyebright daily.

Glutathione

Glutathione is already naturally present in the eyes, more concentrated in the lens. It is beneficial because it is a strong antioxidant that can counter the negative effects of free-radical formation caused by the high levels of light and oxygen that enter the eye through the lens. These free radicals are what degrade the proteins in the lens, causing cataracts to form. So if glutathione is present in the lens, it helps in the prevention of cataracts.

Higher levels of glutathione can be found in such foods as almonds, walnuts, and avocados. When used in combination with alpha lipoic acid, glutathione can virtually halt the progress of cataract development. I recommend 50 milligrams of glutathione a day.

Alpha lipoic acid

Alpha lipoic acid works well in concert with glutathione because it helps to replace that antioxidant in the lens of the eye. Alpha lipoic acid is known as the universal antioxidant because it is both fat and water soluble. It can be absorbed by the fatty areas surrounding the optic nerve endings, and it can penetrate the water-soluble areas such as the eye lens. Therefore, it is a very important supplement for the protection of good vision. One hundred milligrams should be taken daily.

Quercetin

Quercetin is found in such foods as onions and apples and in some tea products. Its usefulness has been proven in decreasing cataracts, retinopathy, and inflammation in the eye. It also counters mucus production, so it is helpful in the treatment of allergies, which often cause watery eyes. A dosage of 50 milligrams daily is sufficient.

Taurine

This amino acid is usually present in very high levels in the retina. It serves as a shield to the small nerve endings present in the macula that transmit the images from the eye to the brain, allowing us to see. If taurine is somehow depleted for whatever reason—genetics, poor diet, or otherwise—the nerves are not properly shielded, and vision problems develop.

Interestingly newborn babies do not have the ability to produce taurine right away, but they receive their supply from their mother's breast milk. If the mother decides to feed her infant with a prepared formula, it must contain taurine or the baby will develop eye problems. Adults can supplement the taurine in their eyes by eating fish or other meat products or by taking 100 milligrams per day in capsule form.

Vitamin C

For the treatment of glaucoma, 2 to 5 grams of vitamin C a day will significantly decrease the ocular pressure in the eye, reversing the progression of the disease and perhaps even preventing blindness.

Vitamin C protects so many parts of the body, but because it is water soluble, it is especially important to the health of the eye lens. Because the lens is not supplied by any blood vessels, any nutrients it gets must be able to disseminate through the liquid portion of the lens. Vitamin C is able to do so, and thus it is very important to the health of the eye. A dose of 300 to 500 milligrams is necessary for the prevention of cataracts. Long-term usage provides the best protection, so start now to reap the benefits of good vision later in life.

ESSENTIAL NUTRIENTS TO PROTECT YOUR EYESIGHT		
Nutrient	**Effect**	**Daily Dosage**
Alpha lipoic acid	Antioxidant that regenerates vitamin C, vitamin E, and glutathione—three powerful antioxidants that help defend the lens, macula, and other eye tissues from free radicals	100 mg
Bilberry fruit powder	A natural source of anthocyanins and flavonoids, both of which are powerful antioxidants that help reduce oxidative stress on the eyes	40 mg

ESSENTIAL NUTRIENTS TO PROTECT YOUR EYESIGHT

Nutrient	Effect	Daily Dosage
Eyebright	Herb used to promote proper eye function and to ease oversensitivity to light	10 mg
L-glutathione	Antioxidant that helps defend the lens, macula, and other eye tissues from free radicals	50 mg
Lutein/ zeaxanthin	The most biologically active carotenoids, especially important for promoting macular health	6 mg
Quercetin	Natural antioxidant flavonoid that helps protect the eyes from damage	50 mg
Taurine	Amino acid that has been shown to reduce oxidative damage to your eyes caused by sunlight, while stimulating your body's ability to remove waste by-products that accumulate in the retina	100 mg
Vitamin C	Essential vitamin and antioxidant that neutralizes free radicals in the lens, macula, and other eye tissues	300–500 mg

CHAPTER 16

FIGHT PROSTATE DISEASE

As the sun went down that evening, all the villagers who had any sick people in their homes, no matter what their diseases were, brought them to Jesus; and the touch of his hands healed every one!

—LUKE 4:40, TLB

MOST MEN SUFFER the *plague* of prostate enlargement as they grow older. I call it a plague because the symptoms it causes bring such aggravation and misery, and the treatments offered by traditional medicine are just as unpleasant—at best. While it is a "natural" phenomenon for the prostate to enlarge with age, because the urethra runs directly through the middle of the prostate, any enlargement causes problems with urination—therein lies the misery. Doctors call this simple enlargement *benign prostatic hyperplasia,* or BPH, which indicates that the cells within the prostate have swollen. Four primary symptoms begin to occur in men who are developing an enlarged prostate gland—all of them unwelcome! Unfortunately enlargement of the prostate is extremely common in men. About 50 percent of men over fifty develop prostate problems. By age eighty, 80 percent of men are displaying symptoms.[1]

SYMPTOMS OF PROSTATE ENLARGEMENT

The first thing that a man might notice is that it begins to take him longer to empty his bladder; his urination is slowing down. This indicates that the swelling prostate is pressing against the urethra and impeding the flow of urine. Second, it becomes harder to cut off the urinary stream, and this causes a dribbling problem that many men start to notice. Third, it becomes harder to start urinating in the first place; and finally, a man finds himself getting up in the night more and more frequently to use the bathroom. I have had patients who literally get up every thirty to forty-five minutes all through the night, every night, to go to the bathroom.

These symptoms can be very frustrating! Not only is it an embarrassing situation for a man, but add to that the fact that he begins to lose sleep, and you have a cause for other health problems due to the stress and sleep deprivation he experiences regularly.

TRADITIONAL TREATMENTS AREN'T FUN!

Generally a man has to reach the point of absolute desperation before he agrees to some of the traditional treatments that are available for prostate enlargement. Many doctors will either freeze or burn out the prostate gland, neither of which is comfortable or pleasant for the patient. One newer, experimental treatment is to concentrate high frequency waves onto the prostate, in essence to microwave it to try to shrink the tissue and alleviate the symptoms!

The most commonly used medical treatment for prostate enlargement is called the TURP. A man gets "turped" when he receives a *transurethral resection of the prostate,* a surgical procedure that slices into the prostate to reverse the inflammation. Most men don't want to submit themselves to the most unpleasant procedure of being "turped." But when symptoms worsen so that it is difficult to empty their bladder when they'd like, when they are getting up in the night every thirty or forty-five minutes, or when they begin to suffer incontinence during the day, they are likely to submit to freezing, microwaving, or being turped, just to get some relief!

NATURAL TREATMENTS FOR PROSTATE ENLARGEMENT

Fortunately God has once again provided for the needs of His children. Within the plant kingdom He has placed natural substances that have proven effective in relieving the symptoms of prostate enlargement. Interestingly the plants that produce these healing substances exist in many different parts of the world. For each culture God has created local, unique compounds that provide relief for this very common and miserable condition.

These healing substances, when combined together, wield a potent punch against the symptoms of prostate enlargement. Let me caution you concerning your personal regimen for taking these natural substances. It is common for many people to practically overdose on a certain nutrient when they read that it might be helpful for their condition. The best thing to do, rather than taking just one substance and going overboard with it, is to properly combine them.

Think about how God set up His plant kingdom. He designed the chemicals within foods, but He never intended for us to just eat one food all the time. God planned for us to have a balanced diet, and He spread out the nutrients through different foods for us to enjoy. As you learn to combine these natural remedies, you can watch the symptoms of prostate enlargement begin to disappear!

(If you are experiencing symptoms of a prostate disorder, see a doctor to ensure your symptoms are not caused by something more serious. If they are not due to a more serious condition such as prostate cancer, I recommend you try some of these natural treatments.)

Saw palmetto

One of the most familiar treatments for the prostate gland is saw palmetto, which works in the body the same way as Proscar, an expensive medication sometimes prescribed to decrease inflammation in the prostate. Saw palmetto naturally inhibits the enzyme 5-alpha reductase, which causes some of the swelling that causes the symptoms. By reducing this inflammation, the prostate gland shrinks and the symptoms are reduced.[2]

Men between the ages of forty and fifty should take 320 milligrams per day, while men over the age of fifty should take 640 milligrams.

Pygeum

Numerous studies have been conducted that show the effectiveness of pygeum, when combined with saw palmetto, in reducing the symptoms of prostate disease.[3] Pygeum actually comes from a plum tree in Africa. A dose of 50 to 100 milligrams of pygeum extract per day is very helpful for men under the age of fifty. Men over fifty should take 200 milligrams a day.

Beta-sitosterol

The sterols are a type of chemical compound that decreases inflammation. Beta-sitosterol is especially effective in decreasing the swelling that occurs in the prostate; therefore, it is particularly good at increasing the urinary flow. Patients who begin taking beta-sitosterol start getting up less and less frequently in the night to urinate. Getting a good night's sleep can make a huge difference in both a man's health and his mood.

Men between the ages of forty and fifty should take 12.5 milligrams per day, while men over the age of fifty should double the dosage to 25 milligrams per day.

Nettle root powder

While it may not sound like a smart idea to put something called *nettle root powder* into your body, nettle root powder has actually been used in many different countries as another potent anti-inflammatory. It not only contains the beta-sitosterol we just discussed, but it also contains several other equally powerful sterols, which shrink the prostate and cause a decrease in the symptoms that men suffer.

Men between the ages of forty and fifty should take 150 milligrams per day, but men over the age of fifty should take 300 milligrams daily.

Rye pollen extract

Rye pollen extract has been used extensively in Europe for several decades. It works in two primary ways. Much like the other treatments we have discussed, it shrinks the prostate gland, bringing symptom relief, but additionally it increases the force of bladder contractions. This helps a man begin to urinate when he needs to, and it prevents many of the dribbling problems that are such an annoyance.

Men between the ages of forty and fifty should take 189 milligrams per day, but men over the age of fifty should take the recommended dose of 378 milligrams daily.

Red clover and soy

Red clover and soy share similar properties due to a common compound they share known as an *isoflavone*. In countries such as China where diets include a lot of soy, both prostate enlargement and prostate cancer are almost unheard of. Red clover actually has four different isoflavones, and soy has two, including the most common, *genistein*. But when red clover and soy are taken together, the combination of these isoflavones seems to provide protection from inflammation or other problems in the prostate.

Men between the ages of forty and fifty should take 80 milligrams of red clover blossom extract and 12.5 milligrams of soy isoflavones. Men over the age of fifty should double these dosages to 160 milligrams per day of red clover blossom extract and 25 milligrams of soy isoflavones.

Pumpkinseed extract

When men who consumed large amounts of pumpkinseeds began to notice an increase in their urinary flow, it was discovered that the sterol compounds within these seeds had an anti-inflammatory effect on the prostate gland. Now fortunately the benefits of the pumpkinseed can be achieved without actually having to eat a pumpkin full of seeds! The extract form is available and is just as effective in treating prostate problems. Men between the ages of forty and fifty should take 10 milligrams of pumpkinseed powder; men over the age of fifty should take 20 milligrams per day.

SEEK EARLY TREATMENT!

So many men put off treating prostate enlargement because of fear or shame until they can hardly empty their bladders! When the condition reaches that point, they could easily end up needing to get "turped." But if the problem can be identified in its early stages, these natural treatments can eliminate the symptoms and the need for unnecessary and unpleasant medical intervention. Women, if your husbands have a prostate problem they are trying to ignore, encourage them to seek help early rather than late. Then make sure they begin taking these natural supplements right away!

God's natural provision is available, but it's up to us to begin to walk in the pathway to healing that He has for us. Pray about the problem, ask God what He would have you do, and then obey His instruction. There is no reason to continue suffering in misery. Begin today to find your pathway to healing of prostate problems.

ESSENTIAL NUTRIENTS TO AVOID PROSTATE PROBLEMS			
Natural Substance	**Effect**	**Dosage for Age 40–50**	**Dosage for Age 50+**
Saw palmetto berry extract	Herb rich in lipids and phytosterols that promote healthy dihydrotestosterone (DHT) levels in the prostate	320 mg	640 mg
Pygeum bark extract	Herb that supports normal hormone levels in the prostate	100 mg	200 mg

ESSENTIAL NUTRIENTS TO AVOID PROSTATE PROBLEMS			
Natural Substance	**Effect**	**Dosage for Age 40–50**	**Dosage for Age 50+**
Beta-sitosterol	Natural plant sterol that promotes healthy DHT levels in the prostate	12.5 mg	25 mg
Soy isoflavones	Source of two key isoflavones—genistein and daidzein—that promote healthy DHT levels in the prostate	12.5 mg	25 mg
Rye pollen extract	Herbal extract containing compounds that promote healthy DHT levels in the prostate	189 mg	378 mg
Nettle root powder	Herb that is a rich source of many phytonutrients—like sterols and lignans—that support healthy prostate function	150 mg	300 mg
Red clover blossom extract	Herb rich in isoflavones that promote healthy hormone levels in the prostate	80 mg	160 mg
Pumpkinseed powder	Natural source of zinc and other nutrients known to be beneficial for healthy prostate tissue	10 mg	20 mg

CHAPTER 17

FIND HOPE FOR PREVENTING BREAST CANCER

*For God has not given us the spirit of fear,
but of power, and love, and self-control.*

—2 TIMOTHY 1:7

THE WORDS BREAST *cancer* strike fear into nearly every woman who hears them. But according to Scripture, God did not give us a spirit of fear. As believers we do not have to live in dread of contracting a life-threatening disease. God promises us a spirit of power, of love, and of self-control. As we pursue His pathway of health and healing, we can be free from fear of disease.

Although nearly 250,000 new cases of breast cancer will be diagnosed this year, and one woman in eight will develop breast cancer over the course of a normal life span, it does not have to strike the child of God. We are not to be frightened or discouraged over these statistics; we have power against this disease through God's revelation knowledge. We not only have spiritual authority through Christ as believers, but we also have God's healing provision in the plant kingdom that will give us power over breast cancer.

TWELVE NATURAL PREVENTIVE MEASURES

The National Cancer Institute has estimated that simply making changes in dietary intake might prevent many breast cancer cases. What follows are the top twelve ways you can keep yourself from becoming a breast cancer statistic.

1. Eat that tofu!

The incidence of breast cancer in Asia, the Mediterranean countries, and numerous other areas in the world are very low. Researchers believe the low rates of breast cancer are due, in large part, to the intake of soy products, as we have mentioned. More recently, as Asians began following a Western-type diet, their incidence of breast cancer rose steadily. The phytoestrogens, known as isoflavones, in soy are actually cancer preventives. These isoflavones bind to estrogen receptor sites and actually guard against the development of breast cancer.

Soy products contain other natural chemicals such as *protease inhibitors*, which prevent cancer-promoting genes from being activated, and *saponins*, which can keep cancer cells from multiplying.

Soy can be obtained as a soy-protein powder and used in drinks; soy flour is also available. Of course, the traditional soy dishes—such as tofu—are very healthful, although I have never been a big tofu fan. Soy products that are fortified with calcium can help prevent breast cancer cells from multiplying and dividing. You might consider trying soy milk on cereal.

2. Take red clover extract.

Perhaps an even better source of these beneficial isoflavones is an extract derived from red clover. Red clover contains four major isoflavones that, when taken daily, appear to be a promising and effective method for women to protect their bodies against the potential of breast cancer.

3. Eat lots of fish.

Study after study demonstrates that women who eat more fish have lower rates of breast cancer. Part of this protection comes from omega-3 fatty acids that are found in fish such as salmon, cod, mackerel, herring, sardines, and trout. The omega-3 fatty acids are really oils that the human body can convert to a chemical known as *prostaglandins*. Certain types of protective prostaglandins keep breast cells from multiplying and dividing.

Patients with a strong family history of breast cancer or unusually thick breasts with increased amounts of fibrous tissue might want to consider taking omega-3 capsules daily. A study published in the *Journal of the National Cancer Institute* found that taking fish oil capsules increased the concentration of omega-3 fatty acids (EPA and DHA) in breast tissue. A higher ratio of omega-3 fatty acids to omega-6 fatty acids is linked to a lower risk of developing breast cancer.[1] Some natural sources are canola oil, walnuts, and flaxseed.

4. Avoid cooking with corn oil.

Certain types of oils, such as saturated fats and other vegetable oils containing omega-6 fatty acids, may actually promote breast cancer. Polyunsaturated oils, such as corn oil, may contribute to this also.

5. Add kiwi fruit to your diet.

The *Journal of the American College of Nutrition* ranked kiwi fruit as the most nutrient-dense of all fruits, providing vitamin E, magnesium, and potassium and also proving to be a good source of dietary fiber. Kiwi provides twice as much vitamin C as an orange! Studies show that vitamin C can inhibit breast cell division, thus reducing the risk of breast cancer.

6. Eat ten almonds and five prunes a day.

For some time we have recommended adding nuts to your daily dietary intake. Approximately ten salt-free almonds a day can offer numerous health benefits. Because they are a rich source of vitamin E, they also play an important role in preventing breast cancer.

Laboratory studies show that vitamin E decreases the incidence of mammary tumors that form after exposure to cancer-causing substances. It actually prevented the cancer cells from developing and provided a killing effect on the cells after they developed. A 2015 study published in *Gynecologic and Obstetric Investigation* showed that eating a large amount of seeds or nuts, including almonds, throughout your life can help prevent breast cancer.[2]

Personally, I like to combine the almonds I eat each day with five prunes. Prunes have turned out to be a medical "super fruit" in the fight against cancer. Because of the prune's remarkable ability to absorb oxygen free radicals, they may also help retard the aging process in the body, especially in the brain.

7. Go orange.

There are some unique chemicals contained in citrus fruits, and especially in oranges, that fight breast cancer. *Hesperetin* and *naringenin* both prevent cancer cell division and also help neutralize cancer-causing chemicals in the body. Another chemical found in oranges, *limonene*, has potent cancer-fighting properties.

8. Take psyllium.

Add 1 tablespoon of psyllium to your diet daily, and you can further lower your risk of breast cancer. Women who eat more dietary fiber have a lower risk of breast cancer than those who eat less fiber. Consumption of psyllium and wheat bran results in a much lower rate of tumor development. You can buy psyllium husks or orange-flavored psyllium supplements (which I prefer) and use them daily in your diet.

9. Fiber, fiber, fiber.

Fibers such as wheat bran tend to bind cancer-causing agents in the gastrointestinal tract and keep them from being absorbed. While psyllium is one good source of fiber, there are others. These sources of fiber include fruits and vegetables in general, and particularly the skin or peels of fruits such as apples. Pinto beans are also a good fiber source, as are kidney beans. When shopping for flour or bread products, look for whole-wheat products.

10. Eat cabbage and broccoli.

God created a unique chemical compound, indole-3-carbinol, that reduces the body's production of certain types of estrogen that lead to breast cancer. I found that these indoles also stop human breast cancer cells dead in their tracks. To reap the benefits of this protective substance, you should eat plenty of cabbage, broccoli, and brussels sprouts.

11. Stock up on yogurt.

Yogurt contains high amounts of calcium, which can inhibit the division of breast cancer cells. Yogurt also stimulates gamma interferon, which helps fight cancer by enhancing the function of the immune system.[3] Multiple studies have shown that dairy, and yogurt in particular, can lower the risk of developing breast cancer.[4] Make sure to eat fat-free yogurt with live cultures but no added sugar or additives.

12. Take vitamin A.

Beta-carotene is the best source of vitamin A. A dose of 15 milligrams daily as a supplement is recommended. Studies consistently show that populations that consume the most vitamin A have the lowest levels of breast cancer.

CHAPTER 18

PMS: STOP THE MONTHLY PLAGUE

He personally carried our sins in his body on the cross so that we can be dead to sin and live for what is right. By his wounds you are healed.

—1 PETER 2:24, NLT

WOMEN DO NOT have to suffer from PMS symptoms. As many as 85 percent of women suffer from one or more symptoms of premenstrual syndrome (PMS), according to the American College of Obstetricians and Gynecologists.[1] The most common complaints seem to center around mood symptoms such as irritability, anxiety, or depression that occur in the week or two before menstruation.

Many women suddenly find themselves weeping, screaming with anger and frustration, or feeling unusually tense with no real external cause. Although the exact causes for premenstrual syndrome are not fully understood, researchers suspect that it is the result of a hormonal imbalance and an increased sensitivity to those unbalanced hormones.

The end result of the hormone imbalance is a lowered level of the brain chemical neurotransmitter *serotonin*. Some studies indicate that in women who suffer PMS, the ratio of estrogen to progesterone tends to be higher than in women who are free of PMS symptoms. Certain lifestyle changes are recommended to all women who suffer from PMS, such as decreasing caffeine intake and increasing exercise levels.

NATURAL SUPPLEMENTS CAN HELP

Data are beginning to accumulate on the value of certain supplements as effective treatments for PMS.

Calcium

For years doctors have observed one interesting association that has not been understood. Women who suffered from PMS when they were younger had a much higher risk of developing osteoporosis as they grew older. As it turns out, calcium is probably the common deficiency in both premenstrual syndrome and osteoporosis. Not surprisingly, then, calcium supplements are an effective treatment for the troubling symptoms of PMS.

The most convincing data on the benefits of supplements for PMS consistently point to calcium supplementation. A study of 720 women showed a nearly 50 percent reduction of PMS symptoms after calcium supplementation.[2] Women who take 1,000 to 1,200 milligrams of calcium daily have a significant reduction in premenstrual symptoms. I currently recommend that women (and men as well) supplement their diets with a total of 1,000 milligrams of calcium in four different forms—the citrate, carbonate, ascorbate, and gluconate forms. All of these can be combined and taken in a basic nutrient supplement. Remember, however, it is the citrate form that is the most easily absorbed of all the calcium supplements.

Vitamins and minerals

Some studies have also suggested benefits in taking supplements of magnesium at a dose of 400 milligrams daily and vitamin E at a dose of 800 international units (in its natural form) daily. Vitamin B_6 has also been widely used for PMS, especially due to its preventive benefits against stroke and heart disease; I recommend taking it at a dose of 75 milligrams a day.

Chasteberry

One herbal supplement that can be very useful in alleviating symptoms of premenstrual syndrome is the herb *vitex*, also known as *chasteberry*. Decreased PMS symptoms were noted in 70 to 80 percent of the women who used this herbal supplement, which tends to increase the levels of progesterone in the body in a natural way.[3] Simply follow the directions on the bottle if you sense that God is leading you to try chasteberry.

God created the female body, and He knows exactly how it functions in all its intricacy. If you are suffering the terrible symptoms of PMS, if it is making you miserable—along with everyone around you—begin to pray and seek God's wisdom as to what path He would have you take to find relief. You don't have to waste one single day on cramps, irritable moods, or discomfort! Begin to pray specifically for the serotonin levels within your brain, that they would come into balance, along with the levels of estrogen and progesterone in your body. Pray for the successful absorption of the necessary vitamins and minerals to help ease your symptoms.

Don't stop at just bringing the problem before the Father in prayer.

Do what things you can do naturally to take care of the situation. I recommend that you try the following:

- Get enough rest.
- Try to reduce your stress levels, especially when you sense the onset of symptoms.
- Take a hot bath to ease the cramps.
- Exercise consistently.
- Cut back on caffeine.
- Begin taking supplements of the vitamins and nutrients I have outlined in this chapter.

Once you have done all that you know to do in following your pathway to healing, stand in faith for it and expect God to keep His promise.

CHAPTER 19

BEAT SYMPTOMS OF MENOPAUSE

*And a woman having a hemorrhage for twelve
years, who had spent all her living on physicians,
but could not be healed by anyone, came behind
Him, and touched the fringe of His garment.
And immediately her hemorrhage dried up.*

—LUKE 8:43–44

JESUS LOVED WOMEN. When our Lord walked on the earth, He elevated the status of women, spending quality time with them, ministering to them, and eventually giving them responsibilities and an important position in His church.

Jesus was concerned about the problems that women face. A very touching incident is described in the eighth chapter of Luke. One day a woman with an issue of blood approached Him for healing. Most likely her medical problem was a female one, and the Bible tells us that she had "suffered much under many physicians" (Mark 5:26). But when she touched Jesus, power flowed from His body into hers, and she was healed.

How important it is for us to turn to Jesus and find the healing pathway that He has planned for us! This woman had suffered under medical treatments that did not cure her, but when she turned to Jesus in her desperation, she received the healing she so desperately needed. And when Jesus realized who it was who touched Him for healing, He commended her faith (Mark 5:34).

God is still concerned about the needs of women today. All women who experience the length of life that God has promised them will pass through *menopause*, which signals a drop in estrogen levels and cessation of fertility. In my clinical research I find that approximately forty-nine hundred women a day enter menopause in this country alone. Menopause is a natural process, but especially in the United States it has become fraught with aggravating symptoms that are difficult to deal with, not to mention the increased possibility of contracting several devastating diseases.

SUFFERING AT THE HANDS OF DOCTORS

In the early 1900s most women would only live to the age of forty-seven or forty-eight, and so menopause was a very rare occurrence. Women simply didn't live long enough to go through it! But as the life span of women began to increase, doctors began seeing certain symptoms appearing in aging women: hot flashes, mood swings, depression, anxiety, and sleeplessness. Unfortunately these symptoms were grossly misunderstood by the medical community.

When a woman who was sitting in a perfectly cool room suddenly broke out into a sweat, or when she sobbed uncontrollably for days at a time, doctors diagnosed it as the only thing they understood it to be: insanity. Many menopausal women were hospitalized in psychiatric units simply for displaying what we consider "normal" symptoms that greet women as they grow older.

Fortunately in the early 1960s doctors began to understand that menopausal symptoms were caused by the body's ceasing to produce the hormone estrogen. Synthetic, artificial estrogen was then offered to women to alleviate the menopausal symptoms, and amazingly, the hot flashes, the night sweats, and the mood swings all disappeared. But then a startling problem began to take place: uterine cancer rates began to skyrocket. Some statistics even show a leap of 13 to 15 percent in women who took prescription estrogen! Eventually doctors discovered that adding progestin to the estrogen that women were taking helped protect the uterine lining and decrease the risk of uterine cancer. But then the risk of breast cancer seemed to leap sky high.

Now it is important to stress that most doctors are motivated by the desire to help people, but without God's help, they are limited in what they understand and in their ability to help. So it is true that many women have suffered at their hands. When we begin to understand that medical treatments cure hot flashes but cause cancer, it is time to seek God for a better way.

SYMPTOMS OF MENOPAUSE

The most obvious problems that women encounter when they reach a certain age actually begin before menopause, involving the cessation of the menstrual cycle, takes place. The phase in which symptoms occur before menopause is called the *perimenopausal* period. These symptoms can be quite aggravating!

One of the first symptoms will be irregular periods. A woman may have two or three normal periods, and then skip one or two, or a period may come at an unexpected time. Then she may notice stranger symptoms: hot flashes and night sweats are among the most common. She may not be aware of more subtle changes that are taking place: Vascular changes in the eye begin to cause a fuzziness in the vision. Forgetfulness, mood swings, anxiety, and difficulty concentrating signal hormonal changes are happening. Many women experience a crawling sensation on their skin, like an insect is crawling on their arm, but when they look, there is nothing there. Urinary tract infections increase as vaginal dryness increases. And one especially troubling symptom that is caused by a decrease in the female hormones is an increasing loss of scalp hair, along with the development of hair in other parts of the body.

DISEASES ASSOCIATED WITH MENOPAUSE

While these symptoms are very annoying to women, they aren't particularly life threatening. However, there are several diseases that often accompany menopause that are far more serious.

Osteoporosis

Osteoporosis, in which a woman's bones become porous and brittle, is perhaps the most well-known disease associated with menopause. Statistics concerning osteoporosis are alarming. About one in four women over age 65 have osteoporosis.[1] By the time a woman reaches eighty years of age, she could easily have lost almost half of her bone mass *and not even be aware of it!* The most frequent clue that alerts a woman to the fact that she has osteoporosis is a fracture of some sort, perhaps a broken hip or a broken leg.

Many times a woman may think she was injured as the result of a fall, but what happens in many cases is that the fall is actually the result of the injury. A woman may be walking along, and because her bones have become so ravaged by the disease, her hip bone will break, or the bones in her leg will snap, and that is what actually causes her fall. You can imagine how easily it would be for this to take place if a woman has lost almost half of her bone mass!

Estrogen has been proven to halt the progression of osteoporosis and even reverse the disease, especially when it is combined with calcium and vitamin D. But as I have already mentioned, with prescription estrogen, the incidences of breast cancer skyrocket. However, in Asia, both osteoporosis and breast cancer are virtually unheard of, and the differences in their diet, as we will discuss, hold the key for our own health in this area.

Heart disease

Among women between the ages of forty-five and sixty-four, one woman in nine will develop heart disease, but over the age of sixty-five, that number triples to one in three![2] It seems that women are protected from heart disease in their younger years, but by the time they reach their sixties, they have caught up with men in the risk of developing heart problems. Heart disease is actually the number-one killer of women.

Breast cancer

Breast cancer is becoming a concern for more and more women, especially because statistics show that 12 percent of women will develop the disease.[3] Prescription-dispensed estrogen and progestin, while providing relief from most of the other symptoms of menopause, have caused skyrocketing rates of breast cancer, as we mentioned.

What are women to do? Modern medicine seems to be offering only two choices: either suffer through the often miserable symptoms that menopause brings, or put yourself at a much greater risk of developing a deadly disease such as uterine or breast cancer. Fortunately God's health plan offers a better option!

Natural Substances Every Woman Should Take

Man cannot duplicate the benefits of God's creation. There are basic substances found in nature that have been proven to provide relief for women who are experiencing hormonal changes in their bodies. They also serve to protect women from developing the deadly diseases we discussed as they grow older. Symptom relief and protection from disease all in one package, without any known side effects! That is God's pathway for a long and satisfying life for women.

Soy and red clover

The isoflavones present in soy and red clover, shown to be beneficial for prostate enlargement in men, have amazing properties for women as well. Soy, especially as an ingredient in tofu and miso, is an important part of Asian women's regular diet. This is a primary reason why so many Asian women do not experience the terrible symptoms of menopause that most American women do. Soy has two primary isoflavones, genistein being the most prominent, and red clover has four, so when these two are taken in combination with each other, the results are powerful.

While soy mimics the diet of most Asian cultures, red clover contains many of the properties of the legumes found in Mediterranean countries, such as beans and chickpeas. In both of these cultures, menopausal symptoms, osteoporosis, and breast cancer are virtually unheard of.

In addition, soy is what is called a "selective estrogen receptor modulator," which simply means that it blocks the receptor sites that would generally bind with the prescription estrogen and cause either breast or uterine cancer. Studies show that women who are taking higher doses of soy isoflavones demonstrate a 54 percent decrease in uterine cancer.[4] The same is true of heart disease.[5]

The FDA has begun to allow soy to make a "heart protective claim," based on the many studies that show its role in decreasing the LDL (bad) cholesterol and increasing the HDL (good) cholesterol levels. Also, the genistein present in both soy and red clover inhibits the breakdown of bone in the body and stimulates the formation of new bone. Amazingly soy and red clover provide powerful symptom relief from menopause and, unlike traditional medical treatments, do not cause breast or uterine cancer, or heart problems. In fact, they actually *protect* women from these diseases!

Fifty milligrams daily of the soy isoflavones and 500 milligrams daily of red clover leaf extract will bring the greatest benefit.

Black cohosh

When a woman needs symptom relief, she generally needs it *now*, if not *yesterday!* Black cohosh, a phytoestrogen (estrogen derived from a plant), begins to show results within *two weeks' time!* This herb comes from a buttercup plant that was used for centuries by Native Americans to relieve menopausal symptoms. The chemicals within the black cohosh also, like the soy and red clover, bind to the receptor sites and help to prevent uterine or breast cancer.

There are no known side effects whatsoever for those who take black cohosh as a supplement; it is one of the safest but most potent herbs available. I have found a significant improvement in symptoms in nearly 100 percent of the women who took it. Black cohosh seems to alleviate headaches, heart palpitations, depression and anxiety, and vaginal dryness, thus preventing urinary tract infections. It also alleviates dizziness, high blood pressure, and high blood sugar.

A dose of 80 milligrams per day is recommended.

Dong quai (angelica)

Dong quai is an Asian herb that is most helpful when combined with the other treatments we are discussing. Its primary benefits are associated with stopping hot flashes and vaginal dryness. A dose of 300 milligrams per day is best.

Ginseng

Having been used for centuries all over the world, ginseng is used primarily as a treatment for stress. Siberian ginseng will improve the mood and stress relief of a woman, especially when her hormone levels begin to drop off as she grows older. The recommended dose is 200 milligrams a day.

Boron

Boron is a mineral that helps the body absorb calcium and therefore proves helpful in strengthening bone structure and protecting women from osteoporosis. Boron should be taken at a dose of 3 milligrams per day.

Bromelain

Bromelain is helpful to the body for a number of reasons. It is primarily an anti-inflammatory, so therefore it helps to prevent blood clots from forming, as well as providing relief from arthritis and other joint problems. In women facing menopause, it is especially helpful in curbing the edema, or swelling, caused by fluid retention. The recommended dose is 45 milligrams per day.

These substances are, I believe, just the beginning of our discovery of the relief God has already provided to women suffering from the terrible symptoms of menopause. Women may have significant problems in this area as they age, but amazingly, as of this writing, over four hundred estrogen compounds have been discovered in nature. God's way is to provide relief from the symptoms and at the same time provide protection from diseases such as osteoporosis and heart disease. What a healing God we serve! You don't have to suffer through menopause anymore! Begin to trust Him today to reveal the pathway to healing He has just for you.

ESSENTIAL NUTRIENTS TO EASE THE DISCOMFORT OF MENOPAUSE		
Natural Substance	**Effect**	**Daily Dosage**
Red clover leaf extract	Herb rich in isoflavones that help balance hormones, promote healthy bones, and support cardiovascular function	500 mg
Dong quai root extract	Herb traditionally used to support hormonal balance in women	300 mg
Siberian ginseng root extract	Member of the ginseng family traditionally used in both China and Russia to help increase resistance to stress, fatigue, and illness	200 mg
Black cohosh root extract	Herb rich in phytosterols that has been used traditionally to help support hormonal balance in women	80 mg
Soy isoflavones	Natural compounds from soy that help regulate hormone balance and support skeletal and cardiovascular health	50 mg
Bromelain	Enzyme that acts as an anti-inflammatory and can help with edema	45 mg
Boron	Mineral that helps strengthen bones and cartilage	3 mg

CHAPTER 20

DISCOVER FREEDOM FROM DEPRESSION AND ANXIETY

He heals the brokenhearted and binds up their wounds.

—PSALM 147:3, NIV

I N TODAY'S SOCIETY depression is becoming an increasingly common problem. Depression can take the form of anxiety, sadness, and eating disorders—resulting in weight loss, weight gain, sleep disturbances, and numerous other problems. The common denominator to all types of depression in the physical realm is a neurotransmitter brain chemical known as *serotonin*. Literally thousands of studies have shown that adding serotonin to the body can relieve the symptoms of depression and anxious depression, and it can help patients lose weight and normalize sleep patterns.

Because it is not possible to give a person serotonin directly, the traditional medical approach has been to use a class of drugs known as SSRIs (selective serotonin reuptake inhibitors). These SSRIs prevent the reuptake of serotonin in the brain, which logically results in increased levels of serotonin. A decreased level of serotonin frequently causes depression, anxiety, and other symptoms.

In general the SSRIs are safe, and literally millions of prescriptions for them have been used. Drugs in this category include Prozac, Zoloft, Paxil, Celexa, Luvox, and others. As with any drug, there are side effects in certain individuals, but generally they are well tolerated. Rarely, more serious problems occur in which patients experience unusual outbursts of temper and violence. Occasional episodes of nervousness and fatigue have also been observed.

Low serotonin levels are now implicated in a much wider variety of diseases than just depression. Some of these include sleep disorders, binge eating, attention deficit disorders, headaches, PMS, and food and carbohydrate cravings that commonly lead to obesity.

THE SEROTONIN SOLUTION

God created certain chemicals—amino acids—that the body naturally converts to serotonin which can help us achieve an increase in serotonin levels. There are several chemicals in this category, but one that has aroused particular enthusiasm is an extract from a plant seed called *Griffonia Simplicifolia*. This seed contains an important chemical called 5-hydroxytryptophan (5-HTP), which helps to normalize the levels of our critical brain chemical serotonin.

THE WONDER OF 5-HTP

Usually the body uses an amino acid called L-tryptophan to convert to serotonin in the human body. Tryptophan occurs naturally in milk, turkey, and other foods. (This is probably why you get sleepy after eating a turkey dinner or drinking a warm glass of milk at night.) Before tryptophan is converted to the beneficial brain transmitter serotonin, it is first converted to 5-HTP. However, when you ingest 5-HTP directly, as a supplement extracted from the Griffonia seed, 70 percent of it is converted to serotonin, compared to 3 to 5 percent of the tryptophan from the foods you eat.[1]

I have found that 5-HTP helps not only with depression but also with anxiety symptoms. Many patients do not realize that anxiety can be part of true depression, although this seems like somewhat of a paradox. Another benefit is that these neurotransmitter chemicals in the brain can have a direct effect on appetite, and 5-HTP can help overweight patients achieve weight loss. Insomnia, which is also common with depression, also decreases markedly when the patient is on this natural supplement.

5-HTP will often produce results when traditional prescription antidepressants fail. One study involved ninety-nine patients whose conditions did not respond to any attempts at alleviating their depression. They were given the supplement 5-HTP at dosages averaging 200 milligrams daily and ranging as high as 600 milligrams daily. Nearly half of these patients made a complete recovery![2] It would certainly make sense that if 5-HTP works so well in these hard-to-treat patients, it would work even better in the more commonly encountered mild to moderate depression.

In my clinical experience I have found that 5-HTP was equal to or better than the typically prescribed antidepressants. A major advantage was that it not only worked, but also the side effects typically were very mild, with the most frequent being mild nausea occurring in less than 10 percent of all patients. However, because 5-HTP is eliminated through the kidneys, patients with renal disease should avoid 5-HTP, as should those patients with peptic ulcer disease.

There are many other neurotransmitters in the brain that are critically important, including dopamine and norepinephrine. Serotonin appears to be one of the most prominent, and amazingly we now have a God-created chemical that can have a direct effect on the increasingly common problem of depression.

For mild to moderate depression, a dose of 50 milligrams of 5-HTP three times daily for two weeks is a good starting point. The dosage can be increased to 100 milligrams three times daily if improvement is not seen. Coated capsules or tablets are now available, which seem to decrease the nausea that patients might experience.

Weight loss

It has been noted for some time that prescription antidepressants that increase serotonin levels can help certain patients lose weight. Since 5-HTP directly increases serotonin levels, it comes as no surprise that it could function as a weight-loss aid.

Though causes for weight gain and obesity are complex, they may be related in part to a decreased conversion of the common amino acid tryptophan to 5-HTP, which results in lowered serotonin levels. In my experience, supplements of 5-HTP were able to reduce high caloric intake, resulting in weight loss even though the patients made no conscious effort to lose weight.

5-HTP also produced a feeling of satiety (the feeling of satisfaction), which results from normalizing serotonin levels. Patients who were on the 5-HTP supplements tended to get full more quickly and simply were not as hungry. I would recommend starting out at a dose of perhaps 50 to 100 milligrams three times daily, and then increasing the dosage gradually.

Headache relief

Many types of recurrent chronic headaches are now associated with serotonin imbalances. This knowledge has produced a new generation of prescription medications that affect serotonin receptors, such as Imitrex and Maxalt. Because of the effect of 5-HTP on serotonin, there have been several clinical studies performed on headaches, including both tension-type headaches and migraine headaches, and the results have been excellent.[3]

Stopping insomnia

Several studies have shown the beneficial effects of 5-HTP in correcting sleep disorders. It is common knowledge that low serotonin levels can lead to chronic sleep disorders. 5-HTP has helped promote sleep by causing patients to go to sleep more quickly and stay asleep longer. I recommend a dosage of 100 to 300 milligrams forty-five minutes before going to bed at night. It is wiser to start with the lower dose and gradually increase it after about three days.

Weight gain, headaches, and insomnia can indirectly cause depression in and of themselves. 5-HTP provides relief from these problems as well as improving the depression itself; therefore, it is very effective in fighting depression and anxiety.

CHAPTER 21

TREAT ALZHEIMER'S DISEASE AND OTHER MEMORY PROBLEMS

Then your light shall break forth as the morning,
and your healing shall spring forth quickly.

—ISAIAH 58:8

HAVE YOU EVER forgotten someone's name? Lost your car keys? All of us show signs of forgetfulness from time to time, especially as we get older, so where is the line drawn between simple forgetfulness and a symptom of a more dangerous, more frightening prospect—the prospect of Alzheimer's disease or another neurological disorder?

One humorous prescription for determining when forgetfulness has become a serious problem says, "It's not Alzheimer's when you forget where you put your car keys. It's Alzheimer's when you forget what the keys are for!"

The problem of neurological impairment—including Alzheimer's disease, dementia, and severe memory loss—is on the rise. Nearly 10 percent of individuals over the age of sixty-five have Alzheimer's; 5.4 million Americans total suffer from the disease.[1] But you don't have to be among the elderly to have problems in this area; almost everyone over the age of forty has some degree of age-related memory loss (ARML).[2]

Despite this seemingly bad news, it is important to keep in mind that the promises of God are still true and that He still wants to satisfy us with a long life lived in fullness on the earth. God's Word is very reassuring when it comes to the problem of decreasing memory and mental function. Consider the following promises:

> But God has not given us a spirit of fear, but of power and of love and of a sound mind.
>
> —2 TIMOTHY 1:7, NKJV

> For God is not the author of confusion, but of peace.
>
> —1 CORINTHIANS 14:33

Confusion may result in losing your car keys! More seriously, confusion occurs in the mind of the Alzheimer's patient who can no longer remember the names of his precious wife and children. God is saying that confusion is not His way—it's not His plan! He has made a way possible for you to walk in divine health, to maintain a sound mind all of your days.

A Doctor's Test for Alzheimer's Disease

Many people begin to forget little things here and there as they age. This forgetfulness causes them to wonder, "Do I have Alzheimer's disease? Am I going to lose my mind?" The key to determining whether or not the problem is serious is to determine whether or not it is *progressive*.

Let me give you an example. Let's consider Tom, a businessman in his early fifties. One day as he is sitting at his office desk, he looks around for his favorite fountain pen and discovers it is missing. This has happened a few times, and he wonders, "Why do I keep losing this pen?" He finds it a few minutes later, right where he had left it; the pen had simply been misplaced. Tom thinks no further of it until he begins to notice he is forgetting names of acquaintances, and then names of close friends whom he has known for years. Finally one day, to his consternation, he gets into his car and realizes he cannot remember the way home from work.

In the earlier stages of this man's forgetfulness there was no real cause for alarm, but once it became progressive, causing him to forget more and more familiar pieces of information, a more serious problem became obvious.

To determine the cause of a possible problem, doctors use a standard memory test. They will state three words aloud to the patient—such as *run, blue, table*—and then tell the person that they will be asked to repeat those words two minutes later in the conversation. Whether or not the patient can complete this task successfully tells the doctor a great deal about the functioning of the memory centers of the patient's brain.

When the doctor states the words, they are stored as a memory and sent down to the entorhinal area of the brain, and finally to the hippocampus, where longer-term memories are stored. Because Alzheimer's affects these areas of the brain first, it is possible to pinpoint potential early Alzheimer's patients if they fail the test.

However, some degree of forgetfulness can be caused by distraction or a lack of attention at the time the information is given. The distraction prevents the listener from incorporating what was heard and moving it into the memory centers of the brain. For that reason doctors will additionally ask the patient about memories from his or her childhood. If the patient cannot remember these memories either, it is a strong indication that something is causing a serious impairment in the brain. Most early Alzheimer's patients would be able to recall childhood memories, but the majority of them would not be able to repeat the list of words. So doctors work backward to find out where the degree of forgetfulness begins and determine the level of impairment from there.

By the way, can you remember the three words we listed before? If you said, "Run, blue, table," you are right, and your short-term memory seems to be working just fine!

Symptoms of Serious Memory Impairment

There are certain symptoms that neurologists check for when they are considering a diagnosis of Alzheimer's or serious memory impairment. The following symptoms are the most common, which I have listed so that you can be aware of developing problems and take steps to avoid a potential crisis.

Short-term memory loss

As I mentioned previously, when doctors give patients three words to remember and then repeat a few minutes later, the majority of those who later developed Alzheimer's were unable to remember two out of the three.

Problems with simple arithmetic

Alzheimer's patients have great difficulty performing calculations or simple arithmetic in their minds. These are not calculations such as finding the square root of 302. These calculations are the simple addition and subtraction problems that we learned as children, such as two plus five equals seven.

Repetition

Now just because your old uncle Joe likes to retell his famous fishing story over and over about when he caught the biggest bass in the county, it doesn't mean that he is in the early stages of Alzheimer's. But if people repeat the same story over and over again because they can't remember that they just told it five minutes ago, it signals a problem. If a person asks the same question over and over again because they don't remember having asked it moments prior, there is some degree of short-term memory loss that has already developed.

Getting lost in familiar places

If a person has taken the same route home from work for ten years but one day cannot remember which way to go, it is a warning sign; a doctor should probably be consulted.

Poor judgment

This is not the poor judgment that a young person might have when he or she makes bad decisions that are based on immaturity. When people suddenly begin to wear soiled clothing or forget to bathe, they are exercising poor judgment because of their mental state. Another example is when a woman continually forgets to turn off the oven or a man leaves the car running in the driveway because he forgot to turn the motor off.

Forgetting names

Forgetting the names of strangers or one-time acquaintances does not usually signal a significant problem. However, a person has already developed a serious problem when he or she can't remember the name of their aunt or uncle, or their closest friend for thirty years, or that of their own mother or child.

Any one of these symptoms may not be an indication of too serious of a problem, but if more than one symptom begins to manifest, and if there are signs of progressive memory loss, it's time to consider getting some help for the problem.

NATURAL REMEDIES FOR MEMORY LOSS

Until just recently the medical community has believed that once a neuron, a nerve cell, died—including the cells of the brain—it could never be regenerated, or brought back to life. They believed the body could heal itself in every other tissue or organ, but once damage was done in the brain, it was irreversible.

But now scientists have learned that brain cells, or neurons, can and do regenerate under the proper conditions. The following natural substances are proven remedies for improving memory function as well as stopping the progress of the devastating Alzheimer's disease.

Huperzine-A (club moss)

When the brain's nerve cells communicate among themselves, they send signals to the various parts of the body to perform their various functions—the heart to beat, the lungs to breathe, the feet to walk, and so on. This critical communication occurs because of the various chemicals that move in areas between the cells, called synapses. The chemical that communicates memories between these neurons is called *acetylcholine*. As you age, the level of acetylcholine in your brain begins to decrease, and as a result your memory function begins to deteriorate.

In modern medicine there are a number of drugs that serve to increase the chemical acetylcholine in our brains and thus promote good memory—these include Aricept, Cognex, Exelon, and Reminyl—but they are very expensive and, like all man-made drugs, have side effects.

A natural source of the chemical huperzine-A, which amazingly has been found to increase acetylcholine levels just as effectively as prescription drugs, is synthesized from the club moss plant. It inhibits the enzyme that breaks down acetylcholine in the brain, thus allowing the levels to increase. The club moss plant has increased memory, thinking ability, focus, and concentration in many Alzheimer's patients. The recommended dosage is 0.1 milligrams daily.

Interestingly the Chippewa Indian tribe, which lived on the east coast of the United States hundreds of years ago, knew to seek out the club moss plant to improve their memory—*and they sought out the very two species of this plant that increased the acetylcholine levels!* The same can be said for the Chinese culture hundreds of years ago and halfway around the globe. God loves all of His people everywhere, and He has made provision in His creation for all of the nations to be blessed!

Periwinkle (vinpocetine)

For years periwinkle, because of a chemical found in it called vincristine, has been used in traditional treatments for cancer. But about twenty years ago scientists began to learn that another potent chemical in periwinkle, vinpocetine, had helpful properties in dealing with memory loss. Although it is primarily used in Europe, vinpocetine is gaining popularity in the United States. Its primary function in the body is as a vasodilator, meaning that it causes the blood vessels to dilate, or open up, to a greater extent. The reason this improves memory function is that it enlarges the blood vessels to the brain, allowing more oxygen and nutrient supply to the brain.

The human brain is a very selfish organ of the body. Even though it requires only about 2 percent of the space within the body, it demands about 20 percent of the oxygen and the glucose as its primary energy source.[3] Other cells and tissues are able to utilize either glucose or fat, but the brain does not offer this choice. It requires glucose, which must be delivered through the bloodstream.

So when a natural substance works to cause the blood vessels to the brain to enlarge, it increases the blood supply to the brain, which is carrying its vital needs for functioning: oxygen and glucose. When these levels are raised in the brain, the person's memory and concentration will improve, and their absentmindedness and confusion will begin to disappear. One milligram daily is the recommended dose.

Phosphatidylserine (PS)

Phosphatidylserine (PS) is a phospholipid of the human body that is used as the primary building block in the lining of the nerve cell, or nerve sheath, but PS is also present in the soybean plant. When it is added as a supplement to the diet, it can improve failing memory and learning ability in people with ARML (age-related memory loss) in as little as three months!

This improvement takes place because the PS increases and strengthens the membranes of the nerve cells in the brain along which the electrical impulses of communication pass. It also helps glucose, the fuel of the brain, to be absorbed better and thus increase the energy level of the entire brain. When there is better neuron communication and greater brain energy, memory and concentration begin to improve significantly. One hundred milligrams is the recommended daily dose.

Ginkgo

Perhaps the most well-known supplement proven to increase mental function and memory is the extract that comes from the ginkgo tree. Interestingly the ginkgo tree is the oldest surviving species of tree on earth—it even survived the detonation of the atomic bomb in Hiroshima during World War II. Within the leaves of this hardy plant comes a substance that produces amazing results.

One of the primary functions of ginkgo in the body is to dilate the blood vessels and provide a greater flow of oxygen and nutrients to the brain, much like the action of the periwinkle plant. However, because ginkgo also works as a blood thinner, patients who are already on blood thinners such as Coumadin should be careful to take only small amounts of ginkgo. Instead combine it with one of these other listed nutrient remedies and allow God to bring healing to both your blood pressure and your mental functions.

For someone without blood pressure problems, the recommended dosage is 100 milligrams per day.

B vitamins

Vitamin B$_{12}$ has had such a potent effect on preventing the effects of aging nerve cells that it has actually been called the "senility vitamin"! Vitamin B$_6$ is commonly known as a nerve supplement and has been used successfully in the treatment of carpal tunnel syndrome, which is essentially nerve damage in the wrist. This same nerve repair can be done in the brain through a dose of vitamin B$_6$. Folic acid decreases homocysteine levels, but it also signals the body to produce more serotonin, a neurotransmitter that promotes communication among the nerve cells.

Vitamin B$_6$ should be taken at a dose of 6 milligrams per day, while vitamin B$_{12}$ should be taken at 12 micrograms per day. The recommended dose for folic acid is 100 micrograms per day.

Vitamin E

Among people who were taking vitamin E for rheumatoid arthritis, scientists began to find less and less incidence of Alzheimer's disease or other mental difficulties. Eventually it was determined that its anti-inflammatory properties, which were so helpful in dealing with the arthritis, were also helpful in decreasing any slight inflammation within the brain that could impair its functioning. Some other natural anti-inflammatories include curry powder and tart cherries, which are discussed further in chapter 22.

Each of these natural substances can make a great difference in the problem of Alzheimer's disease and memory loss, but the greatest improvements take place when all of these nutrients are allowed to work together in synergy, multiplying their effects.

We are living in a generation like no other generation. Our world is full of pesticides, herbicides, and pollution, all of which take a toll on our bodies—not just our lungs, blood pressure, or immune systems, but on our nerve and brain cells as well. Thank God for His provision through the natural plant kingdom, which gives us a way to protect ourselves!

ESSENTIAL NUTRIENTS TO IMPROVE YOUR MIND		
Nutrient	**Effect**	**Daily Dosage**
Ginkgo biloba leaf extract	Herb that increases blood flow and oxygen transport to the brain and helps brain cells communicate	100 mg

ESSENTIAL NUTRIENTS TO IMPROVE YOUR MIND		
Nutrient	**Effect**	**Daily Dosage**
Huperzine-A	Herbal extract that helps maintain healthy levels of acetylcholine, a key neurotransmitter for learning and memory	0.1 mg
Phosphatidylserine complex	Nutrient that enhances the production of neurotransmitters and helps promote memory function	100 mg
Vinpocetine	Herbal extract that improves memory function by enhancing circulation to the brain	1 mg
Vitamin B_6	Essential vitamin that enhances communication between brain cells and protects the brain by lowering homocysteine levels	6 mg
Vitamin B_{12}	Essential vitamin that improves mental function and protects brain cells by lowering homocysteine levels	12 mcg
Folic acid	Essential vitamin that promotes normal growth and development of nerve tissue and protects brain cells by lowering homocysteine levels	100 mcg

CHAPTER 22

USE NATURAL SOLUTIONS FOR ARTHRITIS

Be not wise in your own eyes: reverently fear and
worship the Lord and turn [entirely] away from
evil. It shall be health to your nerves and sinews,
and marrow and moistening to your bones.

—PROVERBS 3:7–8, AMPC

HURTING EVERY DAY is no way to live. In these days of modern technology, advanced medical techniques, and improved hygiene, we are living much longer than we did just a hundred years ago. Unfortunately many elderly people experience so much pain every day in their bodies that they wish they could just go on to heaven. Although the major killers are still heart disease, cancer, and strokes, arthritis is the leading cause of disability.[1] More than 52 million Americans suffer from arthritis.[2] Between rheumatoid arthritis, osteoarthritis, joint inflammation, and a very painful form of arthritis called gout, it seems that we barely have a chance to avoid it as we age. What is the point of living eighty or ninety years on the earth if the last several decades are filled with debilitating joint pain?

God has provided a plant and animal kingdom full of natural remedies of which we are just becoming aware. After we become Christians we have a renewed spirit man, but we still have to live our lives on Earth in physical bodies. And those physical bodies need to be "renewed" just as our spirits and minds need to be renewed.

ARTHRITIS IS NOT JUST AFFECTING THE ELDERLY

Most of us associate the degeneration of arthritis with something our grandparents had; the idea that younger people could develop arthritis may seem a bit far-fetched. In my experience an astonishing 90 percent of all forty-year-olds have the beginning stages of cartilage degeneration. This does not mean that they are necessarily in pain or are facing disability at that point, but it does mean that without certain changes in their diet and lifestyle, there is a good chance that full-blown arthritis will develop—and not just later in life. Over half of those diagnosed with arthritis are sixty-five years old or younger![3]

What could be the cause of such a trend? First of all, the poor diet that most Americans consume does not contain the nutrition needed to foster healthy cartilage replacement in the joints. Not only that, but the typical diet promotes obesity in our society. And if a person is twenty pounds overweight, this weight-bearing problem is almost certainly causing arthritic changes in their joints, especially the knees and the hips.

Another reason for the growing prominence of arthritis in the younger generation is the increasing number of athletic injuries that occur. If a person has suffered a football injury, a hockey injury, a skating injury, or so on, the risk of arthritis increases sevenfold due to the damage sustained to the cartilage in the joints; as many as 15 percent of individuals with osteoarthritis may have developed it because of a previous injury.[4]

With such alarming risks and such pain and debilitation at stake, thank God that He has made it possible to prevent and even correct the joint pain and worn-out cartilage that causes arthritis. It is becoming increasingly important to take advantage of the preventive measures that God has put in place for us. While Satan would love to keep so many of God's people bound up with the excruciating pain and joint stiffness that arthritis causes, God offers you a better plan.

Below are questions designed to determine if you are exhibiting the signs of arthritis. Answer them as accurately as you can.

1. During the past twelve months have you had pain, aching, stiffness, or swelling in or around a joint?

2. In a typical month were these symptoms present for at least half of the days in the month?

3. Do you have pain in your knee or hip when climbing stairs or walking two to three blocks (¼ mile) on flat ground?

4. Do you have daily pain or stiffness in your hand joints?

5. Are you now limited in any way in any activities because of joint symptoms (pain, aching, stiffness, or loss of motion)?

Your Score: If you answered *yes* to any of these questions, you are exhibiting symptoms that may be arthritis or another condition that needs to be diagnosed. You should confirm this diagnosis with your health care provider.

NATURAL CARTILAGE REPAIR

Since the underlying problem of arthritis involves the disintegration of the cartilage in the joints, the search for symptom relief as well as an ultimate cure involves focusing on three aspects of the cartilage problem:

1. Relief from the pain the destroyed cartilage has caused
2. Control of the inflammation in the joints
3. Regeneration and restoration of the destroyed cartilage

Traditional medicine has made great strides in the first two areas of focus. The first treatment for someone suffering with arthritis is to get their pain under control, and the medical community has devised numerous treatments that give patients effective pain relief. Unfortunately many medical treatments stop at that point.

Traditional medicine's current "breakthroughs" have been taking place in the treatment of the second focus we listed: controlling the inflammation of the joints. You may have seen the deluge of commercial advertisements for medications such as Celebrex. Older anti-inflammatory drugs, including Advil and Aleve, were effective in shrinking the swelling in the joints, but their side effects caused multiple stomach problems, sometimes as severe as ulcers. So scientists went to work and developed a new class of drugs that could counter inflammation effectively without the harmful side effects to the stomach. However, it is still not possible to take such a potent drug as Celebrex or Vioxx without some side effects. Rather than causing simple stomach ulcers, they interact with the kidneys, which can create serious problems for the patient.

The third focus we mentioned—rebuilding the disintegrated cartilage—has not begun to be addressed by the medical community. However, rather than deal with an array of side effects from traditional prescriptions for managing pain and inflammation of arthritis—which can be as bad as or worse than the original problem—many people are exploring the possibility of nutritional supplements for help.

NUTRITIONAL ANSWERS FOR
ARTHRITIS AND JOINT PROBLEMS

The wonderful news is that God has provided elements in nature to help correct these painful arthritic conditions. Some of these nutritional answers provide more than just relief from the symptoms of arthritis;

they can actually *reverse* cartilage damage, restoring health to damaged cartilage caused by the disease—the aspect that traditional medicine has not even addressed.

So what should you do to cope with arthritis if you are suffering from its pain and debilitation? First of all, you should begin to seek God for His pathway to healing for *you*. Consider that your pathway could include the nutrients that God has placed in the plant and animal kingdoms, which have been there since the beginning of time. I encourage you to become acquainted with the following natural resources God has provided that have proven helpful in the treatment of this painful disease.

Curcuma

Curcuma is a substance that comes from turmeric, a plant root commonly found in curry powder. Throughout thousands of years of history, especially in the Near and Far East, people used curcuma to control the pain and swelling in their joints even though they had no idea what its chemical structure or true medicinal value was. I have found that the newer arthritic drugs called Celebrex and Vioxx, which reduce joint inflammation, contain the same active ingredient that is present in curcuma! But better still, curcuma does not create the same kidney problems that these other medications do. I recommend 100 milligrams daily.

Tart cherries

The kind of cherries that create benefits for the joints and cartilage are not Bing cherries or the cherries you would find on top of an ice cream sundae. You would find these beneficial cherries in a cherry pie. They are the tart cherries that most people don't want to eat by themselves because they are so bitter. It is the beneficial chemical in them that causes the undesired tartness. Just as was the case with curcuma, tart cherries have been used for centuries to alleviate arthritic pain and joint swelling.

Researchers at Michigan State conducted a study on these tart cherries and found that the active ingredient used by ancient peoples for thousands of years to relieve their symptoms of arthritis was again *the same ingredient found in the prescription medications Celebrex and Vioxx.* And again, the tart cherries had none of the negative side effects that the prescription drugs did.[5] For these reasons I recommend 100 milligrams a day of tart cherry fruit powder.

Holy basil

Holy basil is another ingredient that contains much of the same properties as curcuma and tart cherries; again, it has been used for hundreds of years to bring relief to painful, swollen joints. One hundred fifty milligrams a day is sufficient to help relieve pain and reduce inflammation.

Boswellia (frankincense)

In biblical times frankincense was a prized possession, so much so that it was among the gifts presented by the Magi—along with such other costly gifts as gold and myrrh—to the very young King Jesus (Matt. 2:11). At that time it was valued primarily for its fragrant aroma, but as people rubbed it on their joints as a perfumed ointment, they began to discover that it had healing properties as well.

Today what was then known as frankincense is called by its chemical name, *boswellia*. Boswellia comes from a plant that contains the active chemical boswellic acid, now proved to be a potent anti-inflammatory substance. Initially the gum resin of the plant was used in Bible days to spread topically on the joints, but today we have discovered that its effectiveness increases when it is taken internally.

In one study conducted on boswellia, out of 150 people given the chemical, 70 percent found that the morning stiffness in their joints disappeared altogether, and a whopping 97 percent noticed a significant improvement in their symptoms.[6] If you are suffering from arthritis, you understand that mornings are often the worst time of day for joint stiffness; as the day begins and you start to move around, the joint stiffness decreases. Boswellia, the frankincense that was presented to our King Jesus, has been shown to cause that morning stiffness to virtually disappear!

How is it able to work so effectively? The researchers found that, again, the same chemical present in the new medications Celebrex and Vioxx are active in boswellia, only, again, *without the side effects!*[7] Two hundred milligrams a day is recommended.

Sea cucumber

A sea cucumber is not a member of the plant kingdom but a marine animal, an underwater creature that feeds on plankton in every sea on earth. As the sea cucumbers, also known as bêche-de-mer, strain the plankton, they collect certain compounds from these tiny marine organisms that have amazing anti-inflammatory properties. Sea cucumber may be taken at a dose of 100 milligrams per day.

Glucosamine and chondroitin

In recent years doctors in the United States have begun to connect with the "nutritional world" in recognizing the healing properties of *glucosamine* and *chondroitin*, especially in the treatment of arthritis. Now the scientific community has been able to witness cases of arthritis where the disease is *actually reversed*.

One study recorded in the medical journal *Lancet* looked at 212 people who suffered from arthritis. Half of them were given glucosamine, and half were given a placebo. The study followed the patients for three years, and the results were amazing. Glucosamine patients showed at least a 25 percent rate of improvement in their symptoms, while the patients on the placebo got worse! Patients receiving glucosamine ultimately lost 80 percent less cartilage than their counterparts![8]

For years doctors considered arthritis a progressive disease, meaning that once a person had it, he knew that his joints and cartilage were on a decline that would continue until his life ended. With the use of glucosamine, however, it is possible to provide patients with a real solution. Glucosamine slows progression of arthritic joint changes.

It works especially well when combined with *chondroitin*, a compound found in animal cartilage. When people take glucosamine without combining it with chondroitin, it can take the glucosamine up to three months longer to "kick in." But when the glucosamine and chondroitin are combined (along with the other natural substances that we discussed), relief can begin to occur within a matter of days. The symptoms will be quickly reduced, and over the long run the disease can be stopped and eventually reversed.

Joint cartilage is a fascinating part of the body. Did you realize that it contains no blood vessels whatsoever? All of its nourishment comes from the fluid surrounding the joint, known as the *synovial fluid*. Each time you take a step, you are literally walking on water because the cartilage that is surrounded by the synovial fluid is actually 90 percent water. When the cartilage wears down and the synovial fluid is depleted, the painful situation occurs in which bone rubs against bone in the joint—especially in the knee and the hip.

To repair this damage, glucosamine works to rebuild the cartilage itself, and chondroitin serves to attract the necessary water to return to the cartilage, inflating like a sponge and building the cushion back up within the joint. Glucosamine should be taken at a dose of 1,500 milligrams a day, and chondroitin at a dose of 100 milligrams a day.

Our God is an amazing God, full of grace and compassion for all of our needs. He has provided a way, within His natural plant and animal kingdoms, for us not only to deal with the symptoms of joint disease but also to know how to repair the damage that was done and restore the joints to the way He intended for them to work. God is in the restoration business!

Bromelain

In the Pacific Islands there is a much lower incidence of joint problems than there is in our own country. That fact may be attributed to their consumption of pineapple. Within the stocky portion of the pineapple, the part that most of us choose not to eat, lies a compound called *bromelain*. It too acts as an anti-inflammatory, decreasing the production of the chemicals in the body that cause swelling. One study showed that bromelain decreased inflammation in up to 60 percent of seven hundred patients who took it in its extract form. And a significant number also reported a dramatic decrease in their pain.[9] An additional study looked at 146 boxers; those boxers who took the bromelain rather than the placebo healed from their bruises and joint injuries three times faster.[10]

Bromelain has other healing properties as well. It can decrease blood clotting and reduce blood pressure, probably because it works as an anti-inflammatory on the arterial walls. For this reason it is beneficial to patients with cardiovascular disease as well as to those with arthritis. Fifty milligrams a day is a sufficient dosage.

Diet and Arthritis

Traditionally doctors have been trained to believe that a person's diet does not affect the progression or severity of arthritic symptoms. That belief is changing. Now, as the medical community is beginning to accept the validity of nutrition's impact on disease and the value of supplementation, we are learning what effect certain nutrients have on disease. For example, the omega fatty acids—specifically the omega-3s, the omega-6s, and the omega-9s—have a direct effect on joint pain and swelling. In fact, if they are taken in the correct balance, these vital nutrients can even reverse the progression of arthritis.

The question has been asked: Can corn oil worsen arthritis? Surprisingly the answer is *yes*. It is a bit ironic that several years ago the American Heart Association recommended that the population change from cooking in saturated fats to cooking with polyunsaturated oils such as corn oil, safflower oil, flaxseed oil, and peanut oil to protect the heart. However, these are all omega-6 fatty acids, which contain a compound called linoleic acid. In the human body linoleic acid is converted into arachidonic acid, which is actually an inflammatory compound—that is, it causes inflammation throughout the body, including in the joints, furthering problems with arthritis and joint swelling and pain.

When the corn oils are *balanced* with the omega-3 fatty acids found in fatty fish, the inflammation caused by omega-6 fatty acids is eliminated. Unfortunately in the typical American diet instead of the correct balance of a one-to-one ratio of omega-6 and omega-3 fatty acids, we have a twenty-to-one ratio! What can be done? First, begin to cut down on your use of corn oil, peanut oil, and flaxseed oil; and second, increase the omega-3s in your diet, either through eating fatty fish or through a dietary supplement.

In conclusion there are three aspects to the battle against arthritis and joint disease:

1. Reduce the pain.
2. Reduce the inflammation.
3. Stop and then reverse the cartilage damage.

Although modern medicine cannot offer viable solutions to all three of these aspects, God in His grace has made all things possible to you through your diligent commitment to seek His pathway for your healing. Choosing to use the substances He created in the plant and animal kingdoms for your use, you can create a battle plan against this disease. You don't have to suffer in pain anymore—begin to take the necessary steps to cure your arthritis and repair your cartilage and joints today!

ESSENTIAL NUTRIENTS FOR CARTILAGE AND JOINT FUNCTION		
Nutrient	**Effect**	**Daily Dosage**
Glucosamine	Nutrient that has been shown in clinical studies to reduce pain and help repair cartilage[11]	1,500 mg
Chondroitin sulfate	Nutrient that works with glucosamine to protect and regenerate joint tissue	100 mg

ESSENTIAL NUTRIENTS FOR CARTILAGE AND JOINT FUNCTION		
Nutrient	**Effect**	**Daily Dosage**
Holy basil leaf extract	Herb that helps relieve pain and reduce inflammation by inhibiting the COX-2 enzyme	150 mg
Turmeric root powder (curcuma)	Herb that helps relieve pain and reduce inflammation by inhibiting the COX-2 enzyme	100 mg
Tart cherry fruit powder	Herb that helps relieve pain and reduce inflammation by inhibiting the COX-2 enzyme	100 mg
Boswellia serrata sap extract	Herb that has been shown to effectively reduce the discomfort of swollen joints and morning stiffness as well as improve grip strength and physical performance	200 mg
Sea cucumber	Natural substance that acts as an anti-inflammatory agent	100 mg
Bromelain	Natural compound that reduces inflammation	50 mg

AUTHOR'S NOTE: If you have renal or kidney problems, you should use caution in taking any kind of herbal medicines, since all orally ingested chemicals go through the liver and are filtered by the kidneys.

APPENDIXES

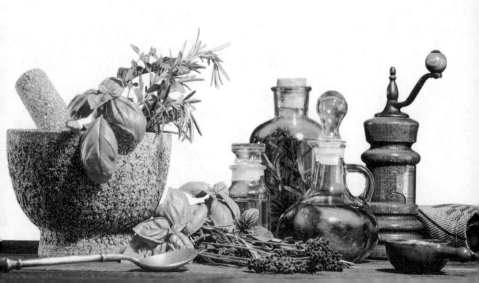

RECOMMENDED DOSES FOR BASIC NUTRIENT SUPPORT

Vitamins and supplements should always be taken with food.

Nutrient	Support Function	Daily Dosage
Biotin	Essential vitamin for healthy skin, hair, and nails	300 mcg
Carotenoid complex	Important group of phytonutrients with antioxidant activity	2,000 mcg
Folic acid	Essential vitamin needed for normal growth and development	600 mcg
Vitamin A (beta-carotene; retinyl palmitate)	Essential vitamin important for the eyes, skin, bones, and immune and reproductive systems	25,000 IU
Vitamin B_1 (thiamin)	Essential vitamin needed for energy metabolism	50 mg
Vitamin B_2 (riboflavin)	Essential vitamin needed for energy metabolism	50 mg
Vitamin B_3 (niacin/niacinamide)	Essential vitamin needed for energy metabolism	100 mg
Vitamin B_5 (calcium pantothenate)	Essential vitamin needed in energy production pathways	50 mg
Vitamin B_6 (pyridoxine)	Essential vitamin needed for amino acid metabolism, neurotransmitter synthesis, glycogen utilization, immune function, and homocysteine regulation	75 mg

Nutrient	Support Function	Daily Dosage
Vitamin B$_{12}$	Essential vitamin needed for proper blood cell formation and cell division	100 mcg
Vitamin C	Essential vitamin needed for its antioxidant activities and for connective tissue repair and regeneration	2,000 mg
Vitamin D$_3$ (cholecalciferol)	Essential vitamin needed for proper calcium metabolism	400 IU
Vitamin E (d-alpha tocopheryl succinate)	Natural, stabilized form of vitamin E that protects cells from free-radical damage	800 IU
Boron	Essential mineral that strengthens bones and supports joint health	2,000 mcg
Calcium	Essential mineral important for bones, teeth, muscles, and nerves	1,000 mg
Chromium	Essential mineral that improves glucose metabolism	300 mcg
Copper	Essential mineral needed for connective tissue, immune function, and nerve cells	2 mg
Hydromins	Natural source of trace minerals essential to life	50 mg
Iodine	Essential mineral needed for proper thyroid function	150 mcg
Magnesium	Essential mineral important for bones, nerves, heart, and muscles	400 mg
Manganese	Essential mineral with antioxidant and connective tissue functions	7.5 mg
Molybdenum	Essential mineral important to many key metabolic pathways	75 mcg

Nutrient	Support Function	Daily Dosage
Potassium	Essential mineral important for fluid balance and nerve cell conduction	99 mg
Selenium	Essential mineral with antioxidant activity	200 mcg
Silica	Essential mineral important for skin, bones, cartilage, and the immune system	7.5 mg
Vanadium	Trace mineral shown to support insulin function and glucose regulation	300 mcg
Zinc	Essential mineral important for skin, bones, cartilage, and the immune system	15 mg
Choline	Essential nutrient that aids in fat metabolism and supports memory function	250 mg
Inositol	Nutrient that supports the health and function of the nervous system	50 mg
Phosphatidylserine	Phospholipid nutrient that supports brain and nerve cell function	100 mg
Fruits and greens powder	Concentrated source of phytonutrients from twenty-four fruits and vegetables	300 mg
Olive leaf extract	Herb that supports cardiovascular and immune function	20 mg
Bioperine	Enhances absorption of a wide range of nutrients	6 mg
Bromelain	Enzyme that aids in protein digestion	50 mg
Cinnamon powder	Herb traditionally used as an aid to digestion	80 mg

Nutrient	Support Function	Daily Dosage
Fennel seed powder	Herb traditionally used to support and enhance digestion	80 mg
Glucono delta-lactone	Promotes healthy growth of beneficial microflora in the intestines	300 mg
Multienzyme complex	Mixture of enzymes that aid in the digestion of carbohydrates, fats, and proteins	50 mg
Papain	Enzyme from papaya that helps with protein digestion	25 mg
Peppermint leaf powder	Herb traditionally used to improve digestion	80 mg
Glucomannan	Soluble fiber that helps curb appetite, regulate blood sugar, and promote cholesterol excretion	150 mg
Alpha lipoic acid	Unique antioxidant and cofactor for energy production	50 mg
Bilberry fruit powder	Natural source of flavonoid and anthocyanin antioxidants	25 mg
Broccoli powder	Natural source of antioxidants and beneficial phytochemicals	50 mg
Cabbage powder	Natural source of antioxidants and beneficial phytochemicals	50 mg
Citrus bioflavonoids	Important group of phytonutrients that enhance the activity of vitamin C	150 mg
Coenzyme Q_{10}	Nutrient essential to energy production in the heart and muscles	25 mg
Glutathione	Important antioxidant and detoxifier in the body	10 mg
Grape seed extract	Natural source of powerful polyphenolic antioxidants	50 mg

Nutrient	Support Function	Daily Dosage
Grape skin extract	Natural source of powerful polyphenolic antioxidants	25 mg
Green tea extract	Natural source of catechin antioxidants	50 mg
Lycopene	Carotenoid antioxidant essential for proper functioning of the prostate	1,000 mcg
N-acetyl-L-cysteine	Important antioxidant and detoxifier in the body	50 mg
PABA (para-aminobenzoic acid)	Nutrient that supports proper cell growth and development	10 mg
Quercetin	Flavonoid antioxidant with anti-inflammatory and antihistamine activity	25 mg
Rutin	Flavonoid antioxidant that supports the strength and integrity of blood vessels	25 mg
Tocotrienol complex	Part of the vitamin E complex with important antioxidant and cholesterol-regulating activity	5 mg
Tomato powder	Natural source of lycopene and other carotenoids	50 mg
Vitamin E (mixed tocopherols)	Part of the vitamin E complex with important antioxidant activity	5 IU
Evening primrose oil	Source of essential fatty acids that support the skin, joints, and immune system	1,000 mg
Marine oils	Natural source of heart-healthy essential fatty acids	2,000 mg

APPENDIX B

RECIPES FOR HEALTHY LIVING

Linda and I have been following the Mediterranean Diet eating plan for several years. Linda has developed many creative, tasty recipes, and we want to share some of our favorites with you.

Cancer-Fighting Lentil Soup

4 Tbsp. extra-virgin olive oil
2 boneless, skinless chicken breasts, all visible fat removed, cubed
12.3-oz. carton firm tofu, cut in cubes
2 stalks celery, chopped
¾ cup shiitake mushrooms, chopped
2 cloves garlic, chopped
1 leek, trimmed of root and green top, chopped
½ cup onion, chopped
½ cup fresh parsley, chopped
½ cup baby carrots, cut in small slices
2¼ oz. sliced black olives, drained
¼ tsp. ground ginger
¼–½ tsp. pure ginseng powder,* to taste
2 14-oz. cans low-sodium, fat-free chicken broth
3 14-oz. cans of water
1-pound bag lentils, sorted and rinsed

In a large soup pot sauté chicken and tofu in olive oil until chicken is white. Remove both from oil and set aside.

Sauté celery, mushrooms, garlic, leek, onion, parsley, and carrots until vegetables are crisp tender. Add black olives, ginger, ginseng, chicken broth, and water. Return chicken and tofu to vegetable mixture. Add lentils. Stir well.

Cook on medium-high heat for 60 minutes or until lentils are tender. Stir occasionally.

Serves 8.

* NOTE: It is important to use American ginseng (Panax quinquefolius). You can search for company names such as CSI Ginseng Products and Pacific Rim Ginseng. Ginseng has an "earthy" and bitter taste; therefore, it is wise to start

with small amounts in cooking and taste-test for desired amounts.

Breadcrumb-Coated Chicken Breasts

1 cup orange juice
1 Tbsp. minced garlic
2 Tbsp. low-sodium soy sauce
1 tsp. olive oil
4–6 boneless, skinless chicken breasts, trimmed of any fat
1 cup whole-wheat breadcrumbs
2 tsp. dried basil, crushed
2 tsp. paprika
¼ tsp. ground red pepper
¼ tsp. ground black pepper

In a 9-by-13-inch nonmetal dish mix orange juice, garlic, soy sauce, and olive oil. Pierce both sides of chicken breasts with fork. Place chicken in mixture and turn to coat both sides well. Cover and refrigerate for 1 hour.

Preheat oven to 350 degrees Fahrenheit. Coat large baking sheet with no-cholesterol cooking spray.

In a shallow bowl mix breadcrumbs, basil, paprika, red pepper and black pepper.

Drain marinade from chicken and discard. Coat chicken well on both sides with breadcrumb mixture. Place on baking sheet. Bake for 20–30 minutes or until chicken is no longer pink in center when tested with sharp knife.

Serves 4 to 6.

Spinach With Apples and Walnuts—a Favorite in France

8 cups fresh spinach, well rinsed
3 Tbsp. extra-virgin olive oil
½ small onion, finely chopped
2 medium to large red delicious apples, peeled, cored, and diced
6 Tbsp. chopped walnuts
Morton Lite Salt and pepper to taste

Place dripping-wet spinach in large pot covered with lid. Cook over high heat for about 3 minutes or until spinach is reduced in volume and slightly softened. Shake pot frequently while cooking without lifting lid. Drain well and press liquid from spinach.

Heat olive oil in large skillet. Sauté onion and apples until onion has softened. (Do not "brown" onion.) Stir in walnuts, and continue cooking for 5 minutes. Add spinach and sauté for 3 minutes longer.

Season with Lite Salt and pepper. Serve immediately. Serves 4 to 6.

Zucchini Pie

2 large eggs, slightly beaten
¼ cup extra-virgin olive oil
¼ tsp. rubbed sage
½ tsp. Morton Lite Salt
¼ tsp. ground black pepper
¾ cup biscuit mix
¾ cup cheddar cheese, 2 percent fat, shredded
1 small onion, chopped
2 cups zucchini, shredded

Prepare a 9-inch glass pie plate with no-cholesterol cooking spray.

In a large mixing bowl slightly beat eggs; then add remaining ingredients in order, stirring to blend well. Pour mixture into pie plate. Bake at 350 degrees for 45 minutes.

Cool for 10 minutes. Slice in pie wedges. Serve with fresh green salad with cherry tomatoes and your favorite fat-free salad dressing.

Serves 6 to 8.

New Potatoes and Green Beans With Pesto

4 cups small new potatoes, washed and cut in half
4 cups fresh green beans, washed and trimmed

Pesto

2 Tbsp. chopped walnuts
1 garlic clove, peeled
3 Tbsp. fresh basil leaves
6 Tbsp. freshly grated low-fat Parmesan cheese
5 Tbsp. extra-virgin olive oil
¼ tsp. Morton Lite Salt
Pinch of black pepper

Boil potatoes for about 10 minutes or until tender.

Boil green beans for about 5 minutes or until tender.

Place remaining ingredients in food processor. Process only until the basil is well chopped (about 10 seconds).

Drain potatoes and green beans. Toss with pesto and serve.

Serves 6 to 8.

Dr. Cherry's Breakfast Cereal Mixture

½ cup Fiber One cereal
⅓ cup oat bran

Combine both cereals in a bowl and add fat-free milk.

Linda's Breakfast Drink

1 package Carnation Instant Diet Breakfast mix
⅓ cup oat bran

Mix together with 10 ounces fat-free (or 1- or 2-percent low-fat) milk.

Strawberry-Banana Milkshake

2 cups buttermilk
1 pint fresh hulled strawberries
2 ripe bananas
Honey to taste

Blend all ingredients in a blender, adding 6 to 8 ice cubes as you blend the mixture. Sweeten to taste with honey.

Oat Bran Muffins

2 cups oat bran cereal
¼ cup brown sugar, firmly packed
2 tsp. baking powder
1 cup fat-free (or 1- or 2-percent low-fat) milk
3 egg whites, beaten slightly
¼ cup honey
2 Tbsp. extra-virgin olive or canola oil

Combine all ingredients. Mix well and pour mixture into 12 muffin cups lined with paper baking liners. Fill muffin cups ¾ full. Bake at 425 degrees for 15 to 17 minutes.

Coleslaw

½ cup Weight Watcher's fat-free whipped salad dressing (or fat-free mayonnaise)
½ tsp. white vinegar
1 Tbsp. extra-virgin olive or canola oil
3 Tbsp. fat-free (or 1- or 2-percent low-fat) milk
2 tsp. prepared mustard
4 packets of NutraSweet (Equal)
1 shredded head of cabbage
2 shredded carrots

Combine all ingredients except the cabbage and carrots. Whip the dressing ingredients with a wire whisk. Pour over shredded cabbage and carrots. Toss until well coated. Serves 6.

Caesar Salad

¼ cup extra-virgin olive oil
1 tsp. lemon juice (fresh or concentrate)
3–4 shakes of red wine vinegar
2 cloves minced garlic
1 squirt anchovy paste
Several sprinkles of freshly ground black pepper
⅓ cup grated low-fat Parmesan cheese
8 romaine lettuce leaves
Tomato or cucumber chunks (optional)

Separate lettuce leaves; rinse in cold water; blot dry; wrap in clean dish towel; and refrigerate for approximately thirty minutes. When ready to serve, tear lettuce into bite-size pieces for salad. Mix all dressing ingredients. Just before serving, pour the dressing over the lettuce and toss well. You may add tomatoes or cucumbers if desired.
Serves 4 to 6.

Tabbouleh Salad

1 cup bulgur wheat
2 cups boiling water
¾ cup minced fresh parsley
¾ cup chopped green onions
¾ cup cooked navy or garbanzo beans
1 cup diced cucumber
2 chopped tomatoes
3 Tbsp. minced fresh mint (or 1 tsp. each dried basil and oregano)
5 Tbsp. extra-virgin olive oil
5 Tbsp. fresh lemon juice
½ tsp. freshly ground black pepper
2 cloves minced garlic
1 small head romaine lettuce

SALAD: In a glass or metal mixing bowl pour the boiling water over the bulgur wheat. Cover the bowl and let it stand for 1 hour. Drain the excess water off the wheat. Add the parsley, onions, beans, cucumber, tomatoes, and mint. Set aside.

DRESSING: Combine the olive oil, lemon juice, pepper, and garlic to make the dressing. Stir the dressing into the salad. Chill for at least one hour. Serve on a bed of whole lettuce leaves. Leaves may be rolled around the salad for eating as a finger food.
    Serves 6–8.

Tomatoes Italiano

2 large halved tomatoes
3 Tbsp. shredded fresh basil (or 1 Tbsp. dried)
1–2 cloves minced garlic
Cracked black pepper
2 tsp. extra-virgin olive oil
Low-fat Parmesan cheese

In a small bowl combine the basil, garlic, pepper, and olive oil. Spread equally on top of tomato halves. Sprinkle lightly with Parmesan cheese. Place in a round glass dish and microwave on high for 3½ minutes. This is good with almost anything.
    Serves 4.

Vinaigrette Dressing

2 Tbsp. red wine vinegar
½ tsp. Morton Lite Salt
½ tsp. dry mustard
6 Tbsp. extra-virgin olive (or canola) oil
1½ tsp. freshly ground black pepper

Combine all ingredients. Whip dressing with a wire whisk until smooth. Pour over chilled lettuce, tomatoes, and other salad vegetables of your choice. Toss until well coated. Serve immediately.

Garlic-Lemon Dressing

½ garlic clove
1 tsp. Morton Lite Salt
1 Tbsp. fresh lemon juice
3 Tbsp. extra-virgin olive oil
Freshly ground black pepper to taste

In a clean, dry salad bowl crush the garlic and salt together with a spoon to make a smooth paste. Add the lemon juice and stir until the salt is dissolved. Add the olive oil and pepper. Mix the dressing well.

This dressing, used in the eastern Mediterranean, is used on green salads as well as over steamed vegetables. It makes ¼ cup.

Low-Fat Lime Dressing

¼ cup nonfat mayonnaise
¼ cup nonfat sour cream
2 Tbsp. honey
2 Tbsp. lime juice
Grated rind from 1 lime
2 cups torn lettuce
2 Tbsp. chopped pecans, almonds, or walnuts

In a cup whisk together the mayonnaise, sour cream, honey, lime juice, and grated rind from one lime.

This is a low-fat, sweet-tart dressing. Serve with seasonal fruit variations. Suggested fruits to use in your own combinations are:

2 cups halved fresh figs
1 cup watermelon balls
1 cup blueberries
1 cup orange sections
1 cup sliced banana
1 cup cantaloupe balls
1 cup diced apple

Other fruits could include raspberries, strawberries, peaches, pears, or pineapples.

In a large bowl toss your chosen fruit combination with one tablespoon lime juice. Let the fruit stand about five minutes to blend the flavors. Place the lettuce on individual plates and top with the fruit and dollops of dressing. Sprinkle with pecans, almonds, or walnuts.

COOKING DRIED BEANS

Rinse 1 pound dried beans in a colander and discard any "bad" beans. Place remaining beans in a pot of cold water. Add 1 tablespoon Morton Lite Salt. Bring beans to a boil, then cover the pot and turn off the heat. Let sit overnight. The next morning, cook the beans until they are tender (several hours), following the directions on the bean package.

There are many ingredients that can be added to beans, including turkey bones that you have saved (keep them frozen until using). Other ingredients include garlic, onions, celery, tomatoes, and cilantro. Herbs and spices that can be added include basil, ground pepper, cumin, oregano, thyme, rosemary, creole seasoning, and other favorites. This is one healthy way to cook beans. Dried bean varieties to use include great northern, navy, pinto, lima, black, and butter beans.

Pinto Beans Deluxe

4–6 cups cooked pinto beans
1 medium chopped onion
1 16-oz. can stewed tomatoes
1 Tbsp. Mexican-style chili powder
1 handful fresh cilantro

Follow the directions on the dried bean package to cook the beans; just before the beans have finished cooking add the onion, tomatoes, chili powder, and handful of fresh cilantro.
Serves 8 to 10.

My Favorite Greens

3 Tbsp. extra-virgin olive oil, divided
1 large chopped onion
2 diced celery stalks
1 bunch collard, turnip, or mustard greens or spinach, OR
1 head of cabbage (core and leaves removed)
1 cup water
Salt-free Mrs. Dash or Parsley Patch

Pour 2 tablespoons extra-virgin olive oil in the bottom of a stainless steel pot. Sauté onion and celery stalks until tender. Place chopped collard, turnip, or mustard greens, fresh spinach, or cabbage in pot. Add the water. Sprinkle the top of the greens with Mrs. Dash or Parsley Patch. Pour 1 tablespoon olive oil on top of the greens. Let cook about 5 minutes. Toss well. Cook on low heat, tossing occasionally until tender.

Serves 8 to 10.

Mediterranean-Style Bean Soup

2 cups dried beans, soaked and drained
2 Tbsp. extra-virgin olive oil
1 large chopped onion
3 medium peeled and chopped carrots
2 crushed garlic cloves
8 cups boiling water
1 14-oz. can stewed tomatoes with juice
1 Tbsp. fresh crumbled thyme (or 1 tsp. dried)
2 bay leaves
Approximately ¼ cup chopped fresh parsley, plus some for garnish
Morton Lite Salt to taste
Freshly ground black pepper to taste
Whole-wheat croutons for garnish (optional)

Soak the beans overnight or prepare according to package directions. In a heavy three-quart stock pot heat the olive oil and sauté the onion, carrots, and garlic until the vegetables are soft but not browned (about 10 minutes).

Add the drained beans and boiling water to soup pot, followed by stewed tomatoes. Then add thyme, bay leaves, and parsley. Cover and cook over low heat 1 to 3 hours, adding water occasionally as needed or until beans are soft (cooking time varies with type of beans).

When beans are soft, add the Lite Salt and pepper. For thicker soup, remove about 1½ cups of beans and purée in a food processor or blender. Return to pot. For thinner soup, add hot water. Garnish with chopped parsley and/or croutons. Experiment by using different kinds of beans each time you prepare this recipe.

Serves 8 to 10.

Linda's Vegetable Soup

1½ onions
1 green bell pepper
½ head of cabbage
3 celery stalks with leaves
4 carrots

Cut the vegetables into medium chunks. Add the following:

1 32-oz. can stewed tomatoes
1 tsp. minced garlic
1 tsp. thyme
1 Tbsp. Morton Lite Salt
½ tsp. freshly ground black pepper
6–8 dashes hot pepper sauce

The following vegetables are optional and could be added to your stock pot before cooking: yellow squash, zucchini squash, fresh brussels sprouts, cauliflower florets.

Combine all ingredients in a large stock pot and bring to a boil. Reduce heat to medium and cook approximately 20 minutes or until the vegetables are tender.

Serves 8 to 10.

Spaghetti Squash

Cut spaghetti squash lengthwise and remove seeds.

CONVENTIONAL OVEN METHOD: Bake squash, cut side down, in shallow baking dish sprayed with olive oil or canola no-stick cooking spray at 350 degrees for 45 minutes.

MICROWAVE OVEN METHOD: Place squash, cut side down, in shallow baking dish with ¼ cup water. Cover with clear plastic wrap. Make several slits in wrap. Cook on high for 7 to 10 minutes.

Remove from oven. Use a fork to scrape the inside of the squash, creating spaghetti-like strands of cooked squash. Add Morton Lite Salt, freshly ground black pepper, and fat-free margarine, if desired.
Serves 4 to 6.

Eastern Yellow Squash Casserole

½ cup nonfat yogurt
½ cup nonfat cottage cheese
½ cup fat-free egg substitute (or 2 eggs)
¼ cup grated low-fat Parmesan cheese
¼ tsp. dried marjoram
1 cup thinly sliced onions
3 cups thinly sliced yellow squash
¼ cup fresh whole-wheat breadcrumbs

In a small bowl blend the yogurt, cottage cheese, eggs (yes, eggs), Parmesan cheese, and marjoram. Set aside.

Coat a large nonstick frying pan with a no-cholesterol, no-stick cooking spray. Add the onions and cook over medium heat for 5 minutes. Coat a 2-quart casserole dish with the same no-stick spray. Spread ⅓ of the squash slices in the dish. Top with ⅓ of the onions and ⅓ of the yogurt mixture. Repeat the layers twice. Sprinkle top with the breadcrumbs.

Cover with aluminum foil and bake at 375 degrees for 20 minutes. Uncover and bake for 5 minutes, or until the breadcrumbs are golden brown. This simple casserole is excellent with baked fish or baked chicken.
Serves 4 to 6.

BAKED OR BROILED FISH

BAKED FISH: Fresh fish generally takes about 20 minutes to bake. If the fish is cut thick, it may take a little longer. Place fish in a baking dish that has been sprayed with olive oil or canola oil no-stick cooking spray. It is not necessary to turn the fish over while baking.

BROILED FISH: Fresh fish generally takes about 5 to 7 minutes per side to broil. Appearance is the indicator. Place fish in a glass dish that has been sprayed with olive oil or canola oil no-stick cooking spray.

HEALTHY TOPPINGS FOR BAKED OR BROILED FISH: Mrs. Dash or Parsley Patch (salt-free), lemon, Fines herbs, Italian herb seasoning, crushed oregano leaves, freshly ground black pepper, crushed parsley leaves, and creole seasonings (salt-free).

Broiled Salmon Steaks

1 salmon steak per person
Fines herbs or Italian herb seasoning
Olive oil

Place the salmon steaks on a broiler pan or cookie sheet covered with aluminum foil or in a shallow baking dish sprayed with olive oil or canola no-stick cooking spray. Sprinkle the tops of the steaks with Fines herbs or Italian herb seasoning. Put a few drops of olive oil in the center of each steak. Broil on the first side for 5 to 7 minutes. Turn the steaks over, sprinkle with seasoning, dot with olive oil, and broil on the second side for 5 to 7 minutes. Serve immediately.

Serving suggestion: Broiled salmon is good with whole-grain wild rice, cauliflower, squash, or broccoli, and salad.

Alaskan Salmon 'n' Rice

2 cups cooked brown rice
1 can (7¾ oz.) drained salmon, liquid reserved
1 cup chopped onion
½ cup chopped celery
½ cup chopped bell pepper
½–1 tsp. curry powder
3 Tbsp. extra-virgin olive oil
1 10-oz. package frozen chopped broccoli, thawed and
drained, or 10 oz. fresh
Dash of freshly ground black pepper

Cook the brown rice according to package directions. Set aside. Drain and flake the salmon, reserving the liquid. Add enough water to the reserved liquid to total ⅓ cup. Sauté onion, celery, bell pepper, and curry powder in the olive oil. Add salmon, rice, broccoli, and reserved salmon liquid. Mix well. Season with dash of pepper. Spray baking dish with olive oil or canola no-stick cooking spray; spread ingredients in the dish. Cover with aluminum foil and bake at 350 degrees for 25 to 30 minutes.

Serves 4 to 6.

Italian Salmon and Pasta Dinner

2–3 large fresh salmon steaks
1 cup sliced mushrooms
1 cup sliced onions
1 Tbsp. extra-virgin olive oil
1 cup diced tomatoes
¼ cup nonfat chicken broth
Pinch of hot pepper flakes
8 ounces fettuccine noodles, or pasta of choice (wheat, vegetable, or whole-grain pasta is best)
2 Tbsp. minced fresh basil
3 Tbsp. grated low-fat Parmesan cheese

Bake the salmon steaks at 365 degrees for 25 minutes, and then flake them. In a large nonstick frying pan sauté the mushrooms and onions in the olive oil over medium-high heat for 5 minutes. Add the tomatoes, broth, and pepper flakes. Cover and simmer over low heat for 5 minutes. Mix with the flaked salmon.

While you are cooking the salmon ingredients, prepare the pasta. Cook the fettuccine noodles in a large pot of boiling water for 10 minutes or until tender. Drain and place on individual plates or a large platter. Add the salmon mixture and basil; toss well to combine. Sprinkle with the Parmesan cheese.

This is a simple dish to prepare. Serve with a dinner salad or a Caesar salad and fruit for a complete meal.

Serves 4.

Chicken and Green Rice

1 whole chicken
2 cups brown rice
2 14½-oz. cans nonfat chicken broth
3 Tbsp. extra-virgin olive oil
1 diced green bell pepper
2 stalks diced celery

1 medium diced onion
2 Tbsp. parsley flakes
1 tsp. Morton Lite Salt
½ tsp. freshly ground black pepper

Boil one whole chicken and remove the bones. Following the rice package directions, cook the rice in the broth, adding enough water to make 4 cups of liquid.

Pour the olive oil in a skillet. Sauté the bell pepper, celery, and onion until tender. Add the parsley flakes, Lite Salt, and pepper. Combine this mixture with the cooked rice. Add the chicken and mix well. (For variation add 1 to 2 teaspoons poultry seasoning and mix well.) Spray a 9-by-13-inch baking dish with olive oil or canola oil no-stick cooking spray. Spread ingredients in the dish. Cover with aluminum foil. Bake at 350 degrees for 45 minutes.

Serves 6 to 8.

Baked Chicken in a Bag

1 whole chicken
½ cup each of diced celery, onion, and carrots
Low-calorie Italian dressing

Stuff a whole chicken with fresh celery, onion, and carrot pieces. Coat the outside skin with low-calorie Italian salad dressing. Place the chicken in a browning bag and place in a 9-by-13-inch baking dish. Make six half-inch slits in the top of the bag. Bake at 350 degrees for 45 to 50 minutes. Remove the skin before eating.

Serves 4 to 6.

Uncle Charles's Skillet Chicken

1 Tbsp. extra-virgin olive oil
2 uncooked packaged chicken breast fillets
1 medium chopped onion
Freshly ground black pepper

Pour olive oil in a skillet. Add onion. Cut the chicken fillets into cubes and add to the skillet. Sprinkle with freshly ground black pepper. Stir and cook until chicken is white and tender, about 10 minutes. Serve immediately over rice, pasta, or potatoes.

Serves 4.

Healthiest Fried Chicken

Canola oil
1 whole chicken, skinned and cut up
1–1½ cups whole-wheat flour
¼ tsp. Morton Lite Salt
¼ tsp. freshly ground black pepper

Heat enough oil in a skillet to fry the chicken. Combine flour, salt, and pepper in a 1-gallon plastic bag. Shake to mix ingredients. Rinse chicken with water. Place chicken pieces in plastic bag and shake well to coat chicken on all sides. Cook in hot oil until golden brown, turning as needed.

Serves 4 to 6.

Serving suggestion: This chicken is good with corn on the cob, steamed vegetables, salad, and especially good with coleslaw. This is a southern delight!

COOKING NOTE: Whole-wheat flour browns more quickly than white flour. Fry chicken on medium-high heat, turning as needed. Watch carefully to ensure that chicken is done.

HEALING SCRIPTURES

Then God said, "I give you every seed-bearing plant on the face of the whole earth and every tree that has fruit with seed in it. They will be yours for food."

—GENESIS 1:29, NIV

If you diligently listen to the voice of the LORD your God, and do what is right in His sight, and give ear to His commandments, and keep all His statutes, I will not afflict you with any of the diseases with which I have afflicted the Egyptians. For I am the LORD who heals you.

—EXODUS 15:26

Worship the LORD your God, and his blessing will be on your food and water. I will take away sickness from among you, and none will miscarry or be barren in your land. I will give you a full life span.

—EXODUS 23:25–26, NIV

The LORD will keep you free from every disease.

—DEUTERONOMY 7:15, NIV

Moses was 120 years old when he died, yet his eyesight was perfect and he was as strong as a young man.

—DEUTERONOMY 34:7, TLB

Thus says the LORD, the God of David your father: I have heard your prayer; I have seen your tears. I will heal you.

—2 KINGS 20:5

Be strong and let your hearts take courage, all you who wait for and confidently expect the LORD.

—PSALM 31:24, AMP

May he redeem their life from deceit and violence; and may their blood be precious in his sight.

—PSALM 72:14

"Because he loves me," says the LORD, "I will rescue him; I will protect him, for he acknowledges my name. He will call

on me, and I will answer him; I will be with him in trouble, I will deliver him and honor him. With long life will I satisfy him and show him my salvation."
—PSALM 91:14–16, NIV

Bless the LORD, O my soul, and all that is within me, bless His holy name. Bless the LORD, O my soul, and forget not all His benefits, who forgives all your iniquities, who heals all your diseases.
—PSALM 103:1–3

Bless the LORD, O my soul, and forget not all His benefits…who satisfies your mouth with good things, so that your youth is renewed like the eagle's.
—PSALM 103:2, 5

He sent His word and healed them.
—PSALM 107:20

I will lift up my eyes to the hills, from where does my help come?
—PSALM 121:1

I will praise You, for You made me with fear and wonder.
—PSALM 139:14

He heals the brokenhearted and binds up their wounds.
—PSALM 147:3, NIV

My son, do not forget my teaching, but let your heart keep my commandments; for length of days and long life and peace will they add to you.
—PROVERBS 3:1–2

Do not be wise in your own eyes; fear the LORD [with reverent awe and obedience] and turn [entirely] away from evil. It will be health to your body [your marrow, your nerves, your sinews, your muscles—all your inner parts] and refreshment (physical well-being) to your bones.
—PROVERBS 3:7–8, AMP

Don't be impressed with your own wisdom. Instead, fear the LORD and turn away from evil. Then you will have healing for your body and strength for your bones.
—PROVERBS 3:7–8, NLT

My child, pay attention to what I say. Listen carefully to my words. Don't lose sight of them. Let them penetrate deep into your heart, for they bring life to those who find them, and healing to their whole body.... Look straight ahead, and fix your eyes on what lies before you. Mark out a straight path for your feet; stay on the safe path.

—Proverbs 4:20–22, 25–26, nlt

He who does not use his endeavors to heal himself is brother to him who commits suicide.

—Proverbs 18:9, ampc

But he was wounded for our transgressions, he was bruised for our iniquities; the chastisement of our peace was upon him, and by his stripes we are healed.

—Isaiah 53:5

Then your light shall break forth as the morning, and your healing shall spring forth quickly.

—Isaiah 58:8

Heal me, O Lord, and I will be healed; save me, and I will be saved, for You are my praise.

—Jeremiah 17:14

"But I will restore you to health and heal your wounds," declares the Lord.

—Jeremiah 30:17, niv

Jesus went throughout all Galilee teaching in their synagogues, preaching the gospel of the kingdom, and healing all kinds of sickness and all sorts of diseases among the people.

—Matthew 4:23

Great crowds followed Him, and He healed them all.

—Matthew 12:15

They will place their hands on sick people, and they will get well.

—Mark 16:18, niv

So He stood over her and rebuked the fever, and it left her. And immediately she rose and served them.

—Luke 4:39

Now when the sun was setting, all those who had anyone sick with various diseases brought them to Him. And He laid His hands on every one of them and healed them.

—Luke 4:40

As the sun went down that evening, all the villagers who had any sick people in their homes, no matter what their diseases were, brought them to Jesus; and the touch of his hands healed every one!

—Luke 4:40, tlb

Then looking around at them all, He said to the man, "Stretch out your hand." He did so, and his hand was restored as whole as the other.

—Luke 6:10

And a woman having a hemorrhage for twelve years, who had spent all her living on physicians, but could not be healed by anyone, came behind Him, and touched the fringe of His garment. And immediately her hemorrhage dried up.

—Luke 8:43–44

There will be mighty and violent earthquakes, and in various places famines and pestilences (plagues: malignant and contagious or infectious epidemic diseases which are deadly and devastating); and there will be sights of terror and great signs from heaven.

—Luke 21:11, ampc

As he went along, he saw a man blind from birth. . . . he spit on the ground, made some mud with the saliva, and put it on the man's eyes. "Go," he told him, "wash in the Pool of Siloam" (this word means "Sent"). So the man went and washed, and came home seeing.

—John 9:1, 6–7, niv

The thief does not come, except to steal and kill and destroy. I came that they may have life, and that they may have it more abundantly.

—John 10:10

Peace I leave with you, My peace I give to you; not as the world gives do I give to you. Let not your heart be troubled, neither let it be afraid.

—John 14:27, nkjv

Pray in the Spirit always with all kinds of prayer and supplication. To that end be alert with all perseverance and supplication for all the saints.

—Ephesians 6:18

Pray without ceasing.

—1 Thessalonians 5:17

For God has not given us a spirit of fear, but of power and of love and of a sound mind.

—2 Timothy 1:7, nkjv

The effective, fervent prayer of a righteous man accomplishes much.

—James 5:16

He Himself bore our sins in His own body on the tree, that we, being dead to sins, should live unto righteousness. "By His wounds you were healed."

—1 Peter 2:24

He personally carried our sins in his body on the cross so that we can be dead to sin and live for what is right. By his wounds you are healed.

—1 Peter 2:24, nlt

Cast all your care upon Him, because He cares for you.

—1 Peter 5:7

The leaves of the tree were for the healing of the nations.

—Revelation 22:2

NOTES

INTRODUCTION

1. "Diabetes Latest," Centers for Disease Control and Prevention, updated June 17, 2014, accessed January 5, 2017, https://www.cdc.gov/features/diabetesfactsheet/.

2. "National Diabetes Statistics Report, 2014," Centers for Disease Control and Prevention, accessed January 5, 2017, https://www.cdc.gov/diabetes/data/statistics/2014statisticsreport.html.

3. James Anderson et al., "Effects of Psyllium on Glucose and Serum Lipid Responses in Men With Type 2 Diabetes and Hypercholesterolemia," *The American Journal of Clinical Nutrition* 70, no. 4 (1999): 466–473.

4. "Grain Fiber and Magnesium Intake Associated With Lower Risk for Diabetes," *JAMA*, Science Daily, May 15, 2007, accessed January 5, 2017, https://www.sciencedaily.com/releases/2007/05/070514174234.htm.

CHAPTER 3—THE FAITH AND MEDICINE CONNECTION

1. Ciddi Veeresham, "Natural Products Derived From Plants as a Source of Drugs," *Journal of Advanced Pharmaceutical Technology and Research* 3, no. 4 (Oct–Dec 2012): 200–201, accessed November 11, 2016, https://www.ncbi.nlm.nih.gov/pmc/articles/PMC3560124/.

CHAPTER 5—GOD'S NUTRITION

1. "Leading Causes of Death," Centers for Disease Control and Prevention, updated October 7, 2016, accessed November 15, 2016, http://www.cdc.gov/nchs/fastats/leading-causes-of-death.htm.

2. "Foods that Fight Inflammation," Harvard Health Publications, updated October 26, 2015, accessed January 5, 2017, http://www.health.harvard.edu/staying-healthy/foods-that-fight-inflammation.

3. Timothy S. Harlan, "Inflammation," Dr. Gourmet, accessed January 5, 2017, http://www.drgourmet.com/column/dr/2016/051616.shtml#.WG57APkrLct.

CHAPTER 6—THE FALLACY OF FAD DIETS

1. "Health, United States, 2015: With Special Feature on Racial and Ethnic Health Disparities," U.S. Department of Health and Human

Services, 2015, accessed November 11, 2016, http://www.cdc.gov/nchs /data/hus/hus15.pdf#053.

2. Dave German, "Overweight and Obesity: Health Consequences," Healthways, May 24, 2013, accessed November 11, 2016, http://health ways.cc/overweight-and-obesity-health-consequences/.

3. Paige Bierma, "Arthritis and Your Weight," HealthDay, updated January 20, 2016, accessed November 11, 2016, https://consumer.health day.com/encyclopedia/arthritis-3/arthritis-management-news-40/arthritis -and-your-weight-644353.html; Deborah Kotz, "Gaining a Pound a Year After Age 20 Nearly Doubles Women's Breast Cancer Risk," US News and World Report, April 20, 2010, accessed November 11, 2016, http://health .usnews.com/health-news/diet-fitness/cancer/articles/2010/04/20/gaining -a-pound-a-year-after-age-20-nearly-doubles-womens-breast-cancer-risk.

4. "Assessing Your Weight," Centers for Disease Control and Prevention, updated May 15, 2015, accessed November 14, 2016, https://www .cdc.gov/healthyweight/assessing/.

5. Go to https://www.cdc.gov/healthyweight/assessing/bmi/adult_bmi /english_bmi_calculator/bmi_calculator.html to find the CDC's BMI calculator.

6. Partnership for Healthy Weight Management, Body Mass Index, retrieved from the Internet at www.consumer.gov/weightloss/bmi.htm.

7. "Nutrition and Weight Management," Boston Medical Center, accessed November 14, 2016, https://www.bmc.org/nutrition-and-weight -management/weight-management.

8. C. J. Henry and B. Emery, "Effect of Spiced Food on Metabolic Rate," Human Nutrition: Clinical Nutrition 40, no. 2 (March 1986): 165–168.

9. "How Lycopene Helps Protect Against Cancer," Physicians Committee for Responsible Medicine, accessed November 15, 2016, http:// www.pcrm.org/health/cancer-resources/diet-cancer/nutrition/how -lycopene-helps-protect-against-cancer.

10. "Metabolism and Weight Loss: How You Burn Calories," Mayo Clinic, September 19, 2014, accessed November 15, 2016, http://www .mayoclinic.org/healthy-lifestyle/weight-loss/in-depth/metabolism/art -20046508.

11. "5-HTP," WebMD, accessed November 15, 2016, http://www .webmd.com/vitamins-supplements/ingredientmono-794-5-htp.aspx ?activeingredientid=794.

12. Rena R. Wing and Suzanne Phelan, "Long-Term Weight Loss Maintenance," American Journal of Clinical Nutrition 82, no. 1 (2005): 222S–225S.

13. M. L. Klem et al., "A Descriptive Study of Individuals Successful at Long-Term Maintenance of Substantial Weight Loss," *American Journal of Clinical Nutrition* 66, no. 2 (August 1997): 239–246.

CHAPTER 7—HEALTHY EATING WITH THE MEDITERRANEAN DIET

1. *Everyday Life in Bible Times*, James B. Pritchard, ed. (National Geographic Society, 1967), 242, 332.

2. "Cancer Mortality and Morbidity," World Health Organization, accessed November 15, 2016, http://www.who.int/gho/ncd/mortality_morbidity/cancer_text/en/.

3. Beth Rice, "Dairy and Cardiovascular Disease: A Review of Recent Observational Research," *Current Nutrition Reports* 3, no. 2 (2014): 130–138.

4. "Study Finds How Red Wine Fights Cancer," *Los Angeles Times*, July 1, 2000, accessed January 19, 2017, http://articles.latimes.com/2000/jul/01/news/mn-46780.

5. "Diet/Nutrition," Centers for Disease Control and Prevention, updated June 16, 2016, accessed November 17, 2016, http://www.cdc.gov/nchs/fastats/diet.htm.

6. Warren E. Leary, "Major U.S. Report on the Diet Urges Reduction in Fat Intake," *New York Times*, July 28, 1988, accessed November 17, 2016, http://www.nytimes.com/1988/07/28/us/major-us-report-on-the-diet-urges-reduction-in-fat-intake.html.

CHAPTER 8—BALANCE THE IMMUNE SYSTEM

1. L. C. Clark et al., "Effects of Selenium Supplementation for Cancer Prevention in Patients With Carcinoma of the Skin: A Randomized Controlled Trial. Nutritional Prevention of Cancer Study Group" [published erratum appears in *Journal of the American Medical Association* 277, no. 19 (May 21, 1997): 1520], *Journal of the American Medical Association* 276, no. 24 (December 1996): 1957–1963.

2. E. Lansky et al., "Further Studies on Pomegranate and Breast Cancer," presented at the IV Madrid Breast Cancer Conference, June 7–9, 2001, Madrid, Spain.

3. Z. Zakay-Rones et al., "Inhibition of Several Strains of Influenza Virus In Vitro and Reduction of Symptoms by an Elderberry Extract (Sambucus nigra L.) During an Outbreak of Influenza B Panama," *Journal of Alternative and Complementary Medicine* 1, no. 4 (Winter 1995): 361–369.

4. Z. Zakay-Rones et al., "Randomized Study of the Efficacy and Safety of Oral Elderberry Extract in the Treatment of Influenza A and B Virus Infections," *Journal of International Medical Research* 32, no. 2 (March–April 2004): 132–140.

5. A. T. Borchers et al., "Mushrooms, Tumors, and Immunity," *Proceedings of the Society for Experimental Biology and Medicine* 221, no. 4 (September 1999): 281–293.

Chapter 9—Diabetes: Starving in the Land of Plenty

1. "2014 National Diabetes Statistics Report," Centers for Disease Control and Prevention, updated May 15, 2015, accessed November 18, 2016, http://www.cdc.gov/diabetes/data/statistics/2014statisticsreport.html.

2. "Diabetes by the Numbers," Stop Diabetes, updated October 24, 2014, accessed November 18, 2016, http://www.stopdiabetes.com/get-the-facts/diabetes-by-the-numbers.html.

3. "The Cost of Diabetes," American Diabetes Association, updated June 22, 2015, accessed November 18, 2016, http://www.diabetes.org/advocacy/news-events/cost-of-diabetes.html.

4. Sue Hughes, "Diabetes Rate Has Doubled Over Past 30 Years," Medscape, June 29, 2011, accessed November 18, 2016, http://www.medscape.com/viewarticle/745494.

5. "Cardiovascular Disease and Diabetes," American Heart Association, updated August 2015, accessed November 18, 2016, http://www.heart.org/HEARTORG/Conditions/More/Diabetes/WhyDiabetesMatters/Cardiovascular-Disease-Diabetes_UCM_313865_Article.jsp/#.WC9bqPkrLcs.

6. "Facts About Diabetic Eye Disease," National Eye Institute, updated September 2015, accessed November 18, 2016, https://nei.nih.gov/health/diabetic/retinopathy.

7. N. Kassaian et al., "Effect of Fenugreek Seeds on Blood Glucose and Lipid Profiles in Type 2 Diabetic Patients," *International Journal for Vitamin and Nutrition Research* 79, no. 1 (January 2009): 34–39.

8. Bolin Qin, Kiran Panickar, and Richard Anderson, "Cinnamon: Potential Role in the Prevention of Insulin Resistance, Metabolic Syndrome, and Type 2 Diabetes," *Journal of Diabetes Science and Technology* 4, no. 3 (May 2010): 685–693.

9. Stephen Daniells, "Science Builds for Cinnamon's Anti-Diabetic Effects," NutraIngredients, April 30, 2010, accessed January 5, 2017, http://www.nutraingredients-usa.com/Research/Science-builds-for-cinnamon-s-anti-diabetic-effects.

10. K. A. Meyer et al., "Carbohydrates, Dietary Fiber, and Incident Type 2 Diabetes in Older Women," *American Journal of Clinical Nutrition* 71, no. 4 (April 2000): 921–930.

11. J. W. Anderson et al., "Effects of Psyllium on Glucose and Serum Lipid Responses in Men With Type 2 Diabetes and Hypocholesterolemia," *American Journal of Clinical Nutrition* 70, no. 4 (October 1999): 466–473.

12. L. Ali et al., "Studies on Hypoglycemic Effects of Fruit Pulp, Seed, and Whole Plant of Momordica Charantia on Normal and Diabetic Model Rats," *Planta Medica* (Stuttgart) 59, no. 5 (October 1993): 408–12; C. Day et al., "Hypoglycaemic Effect of Momordica Charantia Extracts," *Planta Medica* (Stuttgart) 56, no. 5 (October 1990): 426–29; B. A. Leatherdale et al., "Improvement in Glucose Tolerance Due to Momordica Charantia (Karela)," *British Medical Journal* (London) (Clinical Research Edition) 282, no. 6279 (June 1981): 1823–24; A. Raman and C. Lau, "Anti-Diabetic Properties and Phytochemistry of Momordica Charantia L. (Cucurbitaceae)," *Phytomedicine* 2, no. 4 (March 1996): 349–362.

13. S. J. Persaud et al., "Gymnema Sylvestre Stimulates Insulin Release In Vitro by Increased Membrane Permeability," *Journal of Endocrinology* (London) 163, no. 2 (November 1999): 207–12; E. R. Shanmugasundaram et al., "Use of Gymnema Sylvestre Leaf Extract in the Control of Blood Glucose in Insulin-Dependent Diabetes Mellitus," *Journal of Ethnopharmacology* (Limerick) 30, no. 3 (October 1990): 281–294.

CHAPTER 10—BEAT HEART DISEASE

1. "Heart Disease Facts," Centers for Disease Control and Prevention, updated August 10, 2015, accessed November 21, 2016, http://www.cdc.gov/heartdisease/facts.htm.

2. J. R. Berrazueta et al., "The Incidence of Arrhythmias in Young Persons Without Demonstrable Heart Disease: A 24-Hour Holter Study in 100 Medical Students," *Revista Espanola de Cardiologia* (Barcelona) 46, no. 3 (March 1993): 146–151.

3. F. Lopez-Jimenez, "Heavy Meals May Trigger Heart Attacks," American Heart Association Scientific Sessions 2000, November 12–15, 2000, New Orleans.

4. U. Schmidt et al., "Efficacy of the Hawthorn (Crataegus) Preparation LI 132 in 78 Patients with Chronic Congestive Heart Failure Defined As NYHA Functional Class II," *Phytomedicine* 1, no. 1 (June 1994): 17–24.

5. L. Alcocer et al., "A Comparative Study of Policosanol Versus Acipimox in Patients With Type II Hypercholesterolemia," *International Journal of Tissue Reactions* (Geneva) 21, no. 3 (1999): 85–92.

6. Ibid.

CHAPTER 11—LOWER BLOOD PRESSURE—NATURALLY

1. L. A. Ferrara et al., "Olive Oil and Reduced Need for Antihypertensive Medications," *Archives of Internal Medicine* 160, no. 6 (May 27, 2000): 837–842.

2. Ibid.

3. J. C. Witteman et al., "A Prospective Study of Nutritional Factors and Hypertension Among US Women," *Circulation* 80, no. 5 (November 1989): 1320–27; A. Ascherio et al., "A Prospective Study of Nutritional Factors and Hypertension Among US Men," *Circulation* 86, no. 5 (November 1992): 1475–1484.

4. M. R. Joffres, D. M. Reed, and K. Yano, "Relationship of Magnesium Intake and Other Dietary Factors to Blood Pressure: the Honolulu Heart Study," *American Journal of Clinical Nutrition* 45, no. 2 (February 1987): 469–475.

5. "High Blood Pressure Frequently Asked Questions (FAQs)," Centers for Disease Control and Prevention, updated November 30, 2016, accessed January 18, 2017, https://www.cdc.gov/bloodpressure/faqs.htm.

6. Y. Kawano et al., "Effects of Magnesium Supplementation in Hypertensive Patients: Assessment by Office, Home, and Ambulatory Blood Pressures," *Hypertension* 32, no. 2 (August 1998): 260–65; J. C. Witteman et al., "Reduction of Blood Pressure With Oral Magnesium Supplementation in Women With Mild to Moderate Hypertension," *American Journal of Clinical Nutrition* 60, no. 1 (July 1994): 129–35; T. Motoyama, H. Sano, and H. Fukuzaki, "Oral Magnesium Supplementation in Patients With Essential Hypertension," *Hypertension* 13, no. 3 (March 1989): 227–232.

7. N. M. Rao et al., "Angiotensin Converting Enzyme Inhibitors From Ripened and Unripened Bananas," *Current Science* (Bangalore, India) 76, no. 1 (January 1999): 86–88.

CHAPTER 12—FIND RELIEF FROM GASTROINTESTINAL DISORDERS

1. M. H. Pittler and E. Ernst, "Peppermint Oil for Irritable Bowel Syndrome: A Critical Review and Metaanalysis," *American Journal of Gastroenterology* 93, no. 7 (July 1998): 1131–35; J. H. Liu et al., "Enteric-Coated Peppermint-Oil Capsules in the Treatment of Irritable Bowel Syndrome: A Prospective, Randomized Trial," *Journal of Gastroenterology* 32, no. 6 (December 1997): 765–68; M. J. Dew, B. K. Evans, and J. Rhodes, "Peppermint Oil for the Irritable Bowel Syndrome: a Multicentre Trial," *British Journal of Clinical Practice* (London) 38, no. 11–12 (November –December 1984): 394, 398.

2. R. Khanna, J. K. MacDonald, and B. G. Levesque, "Peppermint Oil for the Treatment of Irritable Bowel Syndrome: a Systematic Review and

Meta-Analysis," *Journal of Clinical Gastroenterology* 48, no. 6, (July 2014): 505–512.

3. Dew, Evans, and Rhodes, "Peppermint Oil."

4. M. Camilleri, "Therapeutic Approach to the Patient With Irritable Bowel Syndrome," *American Journal of Medicine* 107, no. 5A (November 1999): 27S–32S; Richard B. Lynn and Lawrence S. Friedman, "Irritable Bowel Syndrome," *New England Journal of Medicine* 329 (December 1993): 1940–1945; Howard Gallagher, *Mayo Clinic Family Health Book* (n.p.: William Morrow & Co., 1996); Lloyd Y. Young and Mary Anne Koda-Kimble, eds., *Applied Therapeutics: The Clinical Use of Drugs, Sixth Edition* (n.p.: Applied Therapeutics, 1995); *Micromedex Healthcare Series* (n.p.: Micromedex, Inc., 2001); Hemant Godara, Angela Hirbe, Michael Nassif, Hannah Otepka, and Aron Rosenstock, *Washington Manual of Medical Therapeutics* (n.p.: Lippincott-Raven Publishers, 1998); Mark R. Dambro, *Griffith's 5-Minute Clinical Consult* (n.p.: Lippincott, Williams & Wilkins, Inc., 1999); Mark Feldman, Bruce F. Scharschmidt, and Marvin H. Sleisenger, eds., *Sleisenger and Fordtran's Gastrointestinal and Liver Disease* (n.p.: W. B. Saunders Company, 1998).

Chapter 14—Treat Headaches and Dizziness

1. A. Grontved et al., "Ginger Root Against Seasickness. A Controlled Trial on the Open Sea," *ACTA Oto-laryngologica* (Stockholm) 105, no. 1–2 (January–February 1988): 45–49.

Chapter 15—Remedy Vision Problems

1. "General Surgery—Common Surgical Procedures," Stanford Health Care, accessed November 21, 2016, https://stanfordhealthcare.org/medical -treatments/g/general-surgery/procedures.html.

2. Dennis Thompson, "Cataract Surgery: A Bargain, Despite the Price," ABC News, accessed November 21, 2016, http://abcnews.go.com/Health /Healthday/story?id=4508775&page=1.

3. J. T. Landrum et al., "A One Year Study of the Macular Pigment: the Effect of 140 Days of a Lutein Supplement," *Experimental Eye Research* (London) 65, no. 1 (July 1997): 57–62.

Chapter 16—Fight Prostate Disease

1. Judy Fortin, "Enlarged Prostate Common in Older Men," CNN, October 22, 2007, accessed November 22, 2016, http://www.cnn.com /2007/HEALTH/10/22/hm.prostate.qa/.

2. L. S. Marks et al., "Effects of a Saw Palmetto Herbal Blend in Men With Symptomatic Benign Prostatic Hyperplasia," *Journal of Urology* 163, no. 5 (May 2000): 1451–1456; Glenn S. Gerber, "Saw Palmetto for

the Treatment of Men With Lower Urinary Tract Symptoms," *Journal of Urology* 163, no. 5 (May 2000): 1408–1412; A. Cristoni, F. Di Pierro, and E. Bombardelli, "Botanical Derivatives for the Prostate," *Filoterapia* 71, Suppl 1 (August 2000): S21–S28; T. J. Wilt et al., "Saw Palmetto Extracts for Treatment of Benign Prostatic Hyperplasia: A Systematic Review," *Journal of the American Medical Association* 280, no. 18 (November 11, 1998): 1604–1609.

3. T. Wilt et al., "Pygeum Africanum for Benign Prostatic Hyperplasia," *Cochrane Database of Systematic Reviews* 1 (2002): CD001044; T. J. Wilt et al., "Phytotherapy for Benign Prostatic Hyperplasia," *Public Health Nutrition* 3, no. 4A (December 2000): 459–472; J. Breza et al., "Efficacy and Acceptability of Tadenan (Pygeum Africanum Extract) in the Treatment of Benign Prostatic Hyperplasia (BPH): A Multicentre Trial in Central Europe," *Current Medical Research and Opinion* 14, no. 3 (1998): 127–139.

Chapter 17—Find Hope for Preventing Breast Cancer

1. Carol J Fabian, Bruce F Kimler, and Stephen D Hursting, "Omega-3 Fatty Acids for Breast Cancer Prevention and Survivorship," BioMed Central, May 4, 2015, accessed January 19, 2017, https://breast-cancer-research.biomedcentral.com/articles/10.1186/s13058-015-0571-6.

2. A. D. Soriano-Hernandez et. al., "The Protective Effect of Peanut, Walnut, and Almond Consumption on the Development of Breast Cancer," *Gynecological and Obstetric Investigation* 80, no. 2 (2015): 89–92.

3. "Super Foods," Cancer Treatment Centers of America, accessed January 5, 2017, http://www.cancercenter.com/community/nutritional-support/super-foods/.

4. Jiajie Zang et al., "The Association Between Dairy Intake and Breast Cancer in Western and Asian Populations: a Systematic Review and Meta-Analysis," *Journal of Breast Cancer* 18, no. 4 (December 2015): 313–322.

Chapter 18—PMS: Stop the Monthly Plague

1. "Premenstrual Syndrome," Office on Women's Health, December 23, 2014, accessed November 22, 2016, https://www.womenshealth.gov/publications/our-publications/fact-sheet/premenstrual-syndrome.html.

2. S Thys-Jacobs et al., "Calcium Carbonate and the Premenstrual Syndrome: Effects on Premenstrual and Menstrual Symptoms. Premenstrual Syndrome Study Group," *American Journal of Obstetrics and Gynecology* 179, no. 2 (1998): 444–452.

3. C. Lauritzen et al., "Treatment of Premenstrual Tension Syndrome With Vitex Agnus Castus Controlled, Double-Blind Study Versus Pyridoxine," *Phytomedicine* 4, no. 3 (September 1997): 183–189.

Chapter 19—Beat Symptoms of Menopause

1. E. J. Mundell, "One in Four Senior Women in U.S. Has Osteoporosis: CDC," HealthDay, August 13, 2015, accessed November 22, 2016, https://consumer.healthday.com/bone-and-joint-information-4/osteo-arthritis-news-42/1-in-4-senior-women-in-u-s-have-osteoporosis-cdc-702230.html.

2. "Heart Disease and Women: How High Is Your Risk?" *The Planned Parenthood Women's Health Letter* 2, no. 3 (May 1995).

3. "U.S. Breast Cancer Statistics," BreastCancer.org, updated September 30, 2016, accessed November 22, 2016, http://www.breastcancer.org/symptoms/understand_bc/statistics.

4. M. T. Goodman et al., "Association of Soy and Fiber Consumption with the Risk of Endometrial Cancer," *American Journal of Epidemiology* 146, no. 4 (August 15, 1997): 294–306.

5. C. M. Hasler, "The Cardiovascular Effects of Soy Products," *Journal of Cardiovascular Nursing* 16, no. 4 (July 2002): 50–63; M. J. Messina, "Soy Foods and Soybean Isoflavones and Menopausal Health," *Nutrition in Clinical Care* 5, no. 6 (November–December 2002): 272–282; L. W. Lissin and J. P. Cooke, "Phytoestrogens and Cardiovascular Health," *Journal of the American College of Cardiology* 35, no. 6 (May 2000): 1403–1410; T. B. Clarkson and M. S. Anthony, "Phytoestrogens and Coronary Heart Disease," *Baillieres Clinical Endocrinology and Metabolism* (London) 12, no. 4 (December 1998): 589–604.

Chapter 20—Discover Freedom From Depression and Anxiety

1. T. C. Birdsall, "5-Hydroxytryptophan: a Clinically-Effective Serotonin Precursor," *Alternative Medicine Review* 3, no. 4 (August 1998): 271–280.

2. L. J. van Hiele, "1-5-Hydroxytryptophan in Depression: The First Substitution Therapy in Psychiatry? The Treatment of 99 Out-patients With 'Therapy-Resistant' Depressions," *Neuropsychobiology* 6, no. 4 (1980): 230–240.

3. Birdsall, "5-Hydroxytryptophan"; G. Bono et al., "L-5HTP Treatment in Primary Headaches: an Attempt at Clinical Identification of Responsive Patients," *Cephalalgia* 4, no. 3 (September 1984): 159–165; G. De Giorgis et al., "Headache in Association With Sleep Disorders in Children: a Psychodiagnostic Evaluation and Controlled Clinical Study—L-5-HTP Versus Placebo," *Drugs Under Experimental and Clinical Research* 13, no. 7 (1987): 425–433.

CHAPTER 21—TREAT ALZHEIMER'S DISEASE
AND OTHER MEMORY PROBLEMS

1. "2016 Alzheimer's Disease Facts and Figures," Alzheimer's Association, accessed November 22, 2016, http://www.alz.org/facts/#quickFacts.

2. Salynn, Boyles, "Memory Loss May Occur as Early as 40," WebMD LLC, January 5, 2012, accessed January 19, 2017, shttp://www.webmd.com /brain/news/20120105/memory-loss-may-occur-40s#1.

3. Amanda Onion, "Studies Show Glucose and Oxygen Help Brain," ABC News, accessed November 22, 2016, http://abcnews.go.com/Health /studies-show-glucose-oxygen-brain/story?id=117530.

CHAPTER 22—USE NATURAL SOLUTIONS FOR ARTHRITIS

1. "Arthritis Facts," Arthritis Foundation, accessed November 22, 2016, http://www.arthritis.org/about-arthritis/understanding-arthritis/arthritis -statistics-facts.php.

2. "Arthritis," Centers for Disease Control and Prevention, accessed November 22, 2016, https://www.cdc.gov/arthritis/.

3. "Arthritis-Related Statistics," Centers for Disease Control and Prevention, updated November 9, 2016, accessed November 22, 2016, https:// www.cdc.gov/arthritis/data_statistics/arthritis-related-stats.htm; "Arthritis Prevalence and Activity Limitations—United States 1990," *Morbidity and Mortality Weekly Report (MMWR)* 43, no. 24 (1994): 433–438.

4. Marie Suszynski, "Post-Traumatic Arthritis: When Old Injuries Come Back to Haunt You," Everyday Health, June 18, 2015, accessed November 22, 2016, http://www.everydayhealth.com/news/when-old -injuries-come-back-to-haunt-you/.

5. H. Wang et al., "Antioxidant and Anti-inflammatory Activities of Anthocyanins and Their Aglycon, Cyanidin, From Tart Cherries," *Journal of Natural Products* 62 (1999): 294–296.

6. V. K. Pachnanda et al., "Clinical Evaluation of Salai Guggal in Patients of Arthritis," *Indian Journal of Pharmacology* 13 (1981): 63.

7. H. P. Amman et al., "Mechanism of Anti-inflammatory Actions of Curcumine and Boswellic Acids," *Journal of Ethnopharmacology* (Limerick) 38, no. 2–3 (March 1993): 113–119.

8. J. Y. Reginster et al., "Long-Term Effects of Glucosamine Sulfate on Osteoarthritis Progression: a Randomised, Placebo-Controlled Clinical Trial," *Lancet* (London) 357, no. 9259 (January 2001): 251–256.

9. S. J. Taussig, "The Mechanism of the Physiological Action of Bromelain," *Medical Hypotheses* 6, no. 1 (January 1980): 99–104.

10. J. L. Blonstein, "Control of Swelling in Boxing Injuries," *Practitioner* 203, no. 214 (August 1969): 206.

11. G. Crolle and E. D'Este, "Glucosamine Sulphate for the Management of Arthrosis: a Controlled Clinical Investigation," *Current Medical Research and Opinion* (London) 7, no. 2 (1980): 104–109; J. C. Delafuente, "Glucosamine in the Treatment of Osteoarthritis," *Rheumatic Disease Clinics of North America* 26, no. 1 (February 2000): 1–11; G. S. Kelly, "The Role of Glucosamine Sulfate and Chondroitin Sulfates in the Treatment of Degenerative Joint Disease," *Alternative Medicine Review* 3, no. 1 (February 1998): 27–39; E. D'Ambrosio et al., "Glucosamine Sulphate: a Controlled Clinical Investigation in Arthrosis," *Pharmatherapeutica* (London) 2, no. 8 (1981): 504–508.

SELECTED REFERENCES

THOUSANDS OF REFERENCES and scientific articles were reviewed for this book, and it is not possible to list them all. You will find listed, however, some of the most relevant and interesting scientific publications that are available at medical libraries. Much of the research was obtained by interviews with research scientists and experts in their fields. In addition news reports from conferences, lectures, and scientific papers were used in the preparation of this book.

"Boswellia Serrata." *Alternative Medicine Review* 3, no. 4 (August 1998): 306–307.

Adlercreutz, H. and W. Mazur. "Phyto-Oestrogens and Western Diseases." *Annals of Medicine* (Helsinki) 29, no. 2 (April 1997): 95–120.

Albanes, D., O. P. Heinonen, P. R. Taylor, et al. "Alpha-Tocopherol and Beta-Carotene Supplements and Lung Cancer Incidence in the Alpha-Tocopherol, Beta-Carotene Cancer Prevention Study: Effects of Base-Line Characteristics and Study Compliance." *Journal of the National Cancer Institute* 88, no. 21 (November 1996): 1560–1570.

Albert, C. M., C. H. Hennekens, C. J. O'Donnell, et al. "Fish Consumption and Risk of Sudden Cardiac Death." *Journal of the American Medical Association* 279, no. 1 (January 1998): 23–28.

Albertazzi, P., F. Pansini, G. Bonaccorsi, L. Zanotti, E. Forini, and D. de Aloysio. "The Effect of Dietary Soy Supplementation on Hot Flushes." *Obstetrics and Gynecology* 91, no. 1 (January 1998): 6–11.

Alvarez-Olmos, M. I. and R. A. Oberhelman. "Probiotic Agents and Infectious Diseases: A Modern Perspective on a Traditional Therapy." *Clinical Infectious Diseases* 32, no. 11 (June 2001): 1567–1576.

Amaducci, L. "Phosphatidylserine in the Treatment of Alzheimer's Disease: Results of a Multicenter Study." *Psychopharmacology Bulletin* 24, no. 1 (1988): 130–134.

Ammon, H. P., H. Safayhi, T. Mack, and J. Sabieraj. "Mechanism of Anti-Inflammatory Actions of Curcumine and Boswellic Acids." *Journal of Ethnopharmacology* (Limerick) no. 2–3 (March 1993): 113–119.

Anderson, R. A., M. M. Polansky, N. A. Bryden, E. E. Roginski, W. Mertz, and W. Glinsmann. "Chromium Supplementation of Human Subjects: Effects on Glucose, Insulin, and Lipid Variables." *Metabolism* 32, no. 9 (September 1983): 894–899.

Anderson, R. A., N. Cheng, N. A. Bryden, et al. "Elevated Intakes of Supplemental Chromium Improve Glucose and Insulin Variables in Individuals With Type 2 Diabetes." *Diabetes* 46, no. 11 (November 1997): 1786–1791.

Arjmandi, B. H., R. Birnbaum, N. V. Goyal, et al. "Bone-Sparing Effect of Soy Protein in Ovarian Hormone-Deficient Rats Is Relevant to Its Isoflavone Content." *American Journal of Clinical Nutrition* 68, no. 6 (December 1998): 1364S–1368S.

Arruzazabala, M. L., S. Valdes, R. Mas, D. Carbajal, and L. Fernandez. "Comparative Study of Policosanol, Aspirin and the Combination Therapy Policosanol-Aspirin on Platelet Aggregation in Healthy Volunteers." *Pharmacological Research* (London) 36, no. 4 (October 1997): 293–297.

Arvill, A. and L. Bodin. "Effect of Short-Term Ingestion of Konjac Glucomannan on Serum Cholesterol in Healthy Men." *American Journal of Clinical Nutrition* 61, no. 3 (March 1995): 585–589.

Aviram, M., L. Dornfeld, M. Rosenblat, et al. "Pomegranate Juice Consumption Reduces Oxidative Stress, Atherogenic Modifications to LDL, and Platelet Aggregation: Studies in Humans and in Atherosclerotic Apolipoprotein E-Deficient Mice." *American Journal of Clinical Nutrition* 71, no. 5 (May 2000): 1062–1076.

Badmaev, V., S. Prakash, and M. Majeed. "Vanadium: A Review of Its Potential Role in the Fight Against Diabetes." *Journal of*

Alternative and Complementary Medicine 5, no. 3 (June 1999): 273–291.

Bai, D. L., X. C. Tang, and X. C. He. "Huperzine A, a Potential Therapeutic Agent for Treatment of Alzheimer's Disease." *Current Medicinal Chemistry* 7, no. 3 (March 2000): 355–374.

Baird, D. D., D. M. Umbach, L. Lansdell, et al. "Dietary Intervention Study to Assess Estrogenicity of Dietary Soy Among Postmenopausal Women." *Journal of Clinical Endocrinology and Metabolism* 80, no. 5 (May 1995): 1685–1690.

Balestreri, R., L. Fontana, and F. Astengo. "A Double-Blind Placebo Controlled Evaluation of the Safety and Efficacy of Vinpocetine in the Treatment of Patients With Chronic Vascular Senile Cerebral Dysfunction." *Journal of the American Geriatrics Society* 35, no. 5 (May 1987): 425–430.

Barnes, S. "Effect of Genistein on In Vitro and In Vivo Models of Cancer." *Journal of Nutrition* 125, no. 3 (March 1995): 777S–783S.

———. "Evolution of the Health Benefits of Soy Isoflavones." *Proceedings of the Society for Experimental Biology and Medicine* 217, no. 3 (March 1998): 386–392.

Barnes, S., C. Grubbs, K. Setchell, and J. Carlson. "Soybeans Inhibit Mammary Tumor Growth in Models of Breast Cancer." In M. W. Pariza, ed. *Mutagens and Carcinogens in the Diet.* New York: Wiley Liss, 1990.

Barnes, S., T. G. Peterson, and L. Coward. "Rationale for the Use of Genistein-Containing Soy Matrices in Chemoprevention Trials for Breast and Prostate Cancer." *Journal of Cellular Biochemistry, Supplement* 22 (1995): 181–187.

Baskaran, K., B. Kizar Ahamath, K. Radha Shanmugasundaram, and E. R. Shanmugasundaram. "Antidiabetic Effect of a Leaf Extract From Gymnema Sylvestre in Non-Insulin-Dependent Diabetes Mellitus." *Journal of Ethnopharmacology* (Limerick) 30, no. 3 (October 1990): 295–305.

Batista, J., R. Stusser, F. Saez, and B. Perez. "Effect of Policosanol on Hyperlipidemia and Coronary Heart Disease in Middle-Aged Patients. A 14-Month Pilot Study." *International Journal of*

Clinical Pharmacology and Therapeutics 34, no. 3 (March 1996): 134–137.

Bendich, A. "Beta-Carotene and the Immune Response." *Proceedings of the Nutrition Society* (London) 50, no. 2 (August 1991): 263–274.

Bennett, J. C., and F. Plum, eds. *Cecil Textbook of Medicine.* 20th ed. Philadelphia: Saunders, 1996.

Berges, R. R., A. Kassen, and T. Senge. "Treatment of Symptomatic Benign Prostatic Hyperplasia With Beta-Sitosterol: An 18-Month Follow-Up." *British Journal of Urology International* 85, no. 7 (May 2000): 842–846.

Berges, R. R., J. Windeler, H. J. Trampisch, and T. Senge. "Randomised, Placebo-Controlled, Double-Blind Clinical Trial of Beta-Sitosterol in Patients With Benign Prostatic Hyperplasia. Beta-Sitosterol Study Group." *Lancet* (London) 345, no. 8964 (June 1995): 1529–1532.

Bielanski, T. E., and Z. H. Piotrowski. "Horse-Chestnut Seed Extract for Chronic Venous Insufficiency." *Journal of Family Practice* 48, no. 3 (March 1999): 171–172.

Bisler, H., R. Pfeifer, N. Kluken, and P. Pauschinger. "Effects of Horse-Chestnut Seed Extract on Transcapillary Filtration in Chronic Venous Insufficiency." *Deutsche Medizinische Wochenschrift* (Stuttgart) 111, no. 35 (August 1986): 1321–1329.

Blumenthal, M., and C. Riggins. *Popular Herbs in the U.S. Market: Therapeutic Monographs.* Austin, TX: The American Botanical Council, 1997.

Blumenthal, M., ed. *The Complete German Commission E Monographs.* Boston: Integrative Medicine Communications, 1998.

Boden, G., X. Chen, J. Ruiz, G. D. van Rossum, and S. Turco. "Effects of Vanadyl Sulfate on Carbohydrate and Lipid Metabolism in Patients With Non-Insulin-Dependent Diabetes Mellitus." *Metabolism* 45, no. 9 (September 1996): 1130–1135.

Bono, G., M. Criscuoli, E. Martignoni, S. Salmon, and G. Nappi. "Serotonin Precursors in Migraine Prophylaxis." *Advances in Neurology* 33 (1982): 357–363.

Bonoczk, P., B. Gulyas, V. Adam-vizi, et al. "Role of Sodium Channel Inhibition in Neuroprotection: Effect of Vinpocetine." *Brain Research Bulletin* 53, no. 3 (October 2000): 245–254.

Borchers, A. T., J. S. Stern, R. M. Hackman, C. L. Keen, and M. E. Gershwin. "Mushrooms, Tumors, and Immunity." *Proceedings of the Society for Experimental Biology and Medicine* 221, no. 4 (September 1999): 281–293.

Breza, J., O. Dzurny, A. Borowka, et al. "Efficacy and Acceptability of Tadenan (Pygeum Africanum Extract) in the Treatment of Benign Prostatic Hyperplasia (BPH): A Multicentre Trial in Central Europe." *Current Medical Research and Opinion* 14, no. 3 (1998): 127–139.

Brichard, S. M., and J. C. Henquin. "The Role of Vanadium in the Management of Diabetes." *Trends in Pharmacological Sciences* 16, no. 8 (August 1995): 265–270.

Brinkeborn, R. M., D. V. Shah, and F. H. Degenring. "Echinaforce and Other Echinacea Fresh Plant Preparations in the Treatment of the Common Cold. A Randomized, Placebo Controlled, Double-Blind Clinical Trial." *Phytomedicine* 6, no. 1 (March 1999): 1–6.

Byerley, W. F., L. L. Judd, F. W. Reimherr, and B. I. Grosser. "5-Hydroxytryptophan: A Review of Its Antidepressant Efficacy and Adverse Effects." *Journal of Clinical Psychopharmacology* 7, no. 3 (June 1987): 127–137.

Byers, T. and N. Guerrero. "Epidemiologic Evidence for Vitamin C and Vitamin E in Cancer Prevention." *American Journal of Clinical Nutrition* 62, no. 6 (December 1995): 1385S–1392S.

Camps, P., B. Cusack, W. D. Mallender, et al. "Huprine X Is a Novel High-Affinity Inhibitor of Acetylcholinesterase That Is of Interest for Treatment of Alzheimer's Disease." *Molecular Pharmacology* 57, no. 2 (February 2000): 409–417.

Canetti, M., M. Moreira, R. Mas, et al. "A Two-Year Study on the Efficacy and Tolerability of Policosanol in Patients With Type II Hyperlipoproteinaemia." *International Journal of Clinical Pharmacology Research* (Geneva) 15, no. 4 (1995): 159–165.

Cangiano, C., A. Laviano, M. del Ben, et al. "Effects of Oral
      5-Hydroxy-Tryptophan on Energy Intake and Macronutrient
      Selection in Non-Insulin Dependent Diabetic Patients."
      International Journal of Obesity and Related Metabolic Disorders
      (London) 22, no. 7 (July 1998): 648–654.

Cangiano, C., F. Ceci, A. Cascino, et al. "Eating Behavior and
      Adherence to Dietary Prescriptions in Obese Adult Subjects
      Treated With 5-Hydroxytryptophan." *American Journal of
      Clinical Nutrition* 56, no. 5 (November 1992): 863–867.

Carbin, B. E., B. Larsson, and O. Lindahl. "Treatment of Benign
      Prostatic Hyperplasia With Phytosterols." *British Journal of
      Urology* (London) 66, no. 6 (December 1990): 639–641.

Castano, G., R. Mas, J. Roca, et al. "A Double-Blind, Placebo-
      Controlled Study of the Effects of Policosanol in Patients
      With Intermittent Claudication." *Angiology* 50, no. 2
      (February 1999): 123–130.

Ceci, F., C. Cangiano, M. Cairella, et al. "The Effects of Oral
      5-Hydroxytryptophan Administration on Feeding Behavior in
      Obese Adult Female Subjects." *Journal of Neural Transmission*
      (Wien) 76, no. 2 (1989): 109–117.

Chandra, D. and S. S. Gupta. "Anti-Inflammatory and Anti-Arthritic
      Activity of Volatile Oil of Curcuma Longa (Haldi)." *Indian
      Journal of Medical Research* (New Delhi) 60, no. 1 (January
      1972): 138–142.

———. "Graying of the Immune System. Can Nutrient Supplements
      Improve Immunity in the Elderly?" *Journal of the American
      Medical Association* 277, no. 17 (May 1997): 1398–1399.

———. "Nutrition and the Immune System: An Introduction."
      American Journal of Clinical Nutrition 66, no. 2 (August 1997):
      460S–463S.

Clark, L. C. and G. F. J. Combs. "Selenium Compounds and the
      Prevention of Cancer: Research Needs and Public Health
      Implications." *Journal of Nutrition* 116, no. 1 (January 1986):
      170–173.

Clark, L. C., G. F. Combs Jr., B. W. Turnbull, et al. "Effects of
      Selenium Supplementation for Cancer Prevention in Patients

With Carcinoma of the Skin. A Randomized Controlled Trial. Nutritional Prevention of Cancer Study Group" [published erratum appears in *Journal of the American Medical Association* 277, no. 19 (May 1997): 1520]. *Journal of the American Medical Association* 276, no. 24 (December 1996): 1957–1963.

Cline, J. M. and C. L. J. Hughes. "Phytochemicals for the Prevention of Breast and Endometrial Cancer." *Cancer Treatment and Research* 94 (1998): 107–134.

Colditz, G. A. and A. L. Frazier. "Models of Breast Cancer Show That Risk Is Set by Events of Early Life: Prevention Efforts Must Shift Focus." *Cancer Epidemiology, Biomarkers, and Prevention* 4, no. 5 (July–August 1995): 567–571.

Crissinger, K. D., P. R. Kvietys, and D. N. Granger. "Pathophysiology of Gastrointestinal Mucosal Permeability." *Journal of Internal Medicine. Supplement* (Oxford) 732 (1990): 145–154.

Crook, T. H. "Treatment of Age-Related Cognitive Decline: Effects of Phosphatidylserine." In *Anti-Aging Medical Therapeutics*, volume II. Marina Del Ray, CA: Healthquest, 1998.

Daviglus, M. L., J. Stamler, A. J. Orencia, et al. "Fish Consumption and the 30-Year Risk of Myocardial Infarction." *New England Journal of Medicine* 336, no. 15 (April 1997): 1046–1053.

De Giorgis, G., R. Miletto, M. Iannuccelli, M. Camuffo, and S. Scerni. "Headache in Association With Sleep Disorders in Children: A Psychodiagnostic Evaluation and Controlled Clinical Study— L-5-HTP Versus Placebo." *Drugs Under Experimental and Clinical Research* 13, no. 7 (1987): 425–433.

De Lourdes Lima, M., T. Cruz, J. C. Pousada, et al. "The Effect of Magnesium Supplementation in Increasing Doses on the Control of Type 2 Diabetes." *Diabetes Care* 21, no. 5 (May 1998): 682–686.

De Simone, C., R. Vesely, B. B. Salvadori, and E. Jirillo. "The Role of Probiotics in Modulation of the Immune System in Man and in Animals." *International Journal of Immunotherapy* 9, no. 1 (January 1993): 23–28.

Deal, C. L. and R. W. Moskowitz. "Nutraceuticals as Therapeutic
    Agents in Osteoarthritis: The Role of Glucosamine,
    Chondroitin Sulfate, and Collagen Hydrolysate." *Rheumatic
    Diseases Clinics of North America* 25, no. 2 (May 1999):
    379–395.

Dew, M. J., B. K. Evans, and J. Rhodes. "Peppermint Oil for the
    Irritable Bowel Syndrome: A Multicentre Trial." *British
    Journal of Clinical Practice* (London) 38, no. 11–12 (November–
    December 1984): 394, 398.

Diehm, C., H. J. Trampisch, S. Lange, and C. Schmidt. "Comparison
    of Leg Compression Stocking and Oral Horse-Chestnut
    Seed Extract Therapy in Patients With Chronic Venous
    Insufficiency." *Lancet* (London) 347, no. 8997 (February 1996):
    292–294.

Doi, K., M. Matsuura, A. Kawara, and S. Baba. "Treatment of
    Diabetes With Glucomannan (Konjac Mannan)." *Lancet*
    (London) 1, no. 8123 (May 1979): 987–988.

Elliott, R. B., C. C. Pilcher, D. M. Fergusson, and A. W. Stewart. "A
    Population Based Strategy to Prevent Insulin-Dependent
    Diabetes Using Nicotinamide." *Journal of Pediatric
    Endocrinology and Metabolism* 9, no. 5 (September–October
    1996): 501–509.

Fraker, P. J., M. E. Gershwin, R. A. Good, and A. Prasad.
    "Interrelationships Between Zinc and Immune Function."
    Federation Proceedings 45, no. 5 (April 1986): 1474–1479.

Fund, W. C. R. *Food, Nutrition, and the Prevention of Cancer: A Global
    Perspective*. Washington, DC: American Institute Cancer
    Research, 1997.

Gandini, S., H. Merzenich, C. Robertson, and P. Boyle. "Meta-
    Analysis of Studies on Breast Cancer Risk and Diet: The
    Role of Fruit and Vegetable Consumption and the Intake
    of Associated Micronutrients." *European Journal of Cancer*
    (Oxford) 36, no. 5 (March 2000): 636–646.

Garland, M., W. C. Willett, J. E. Manson, and D. J. Hunter.
    "Antioxidant Micronutrients and Breast Cancer." *Journal of the
    American College of Nutrition* 12, no. 4 (August 1993): 400–411.

Gerber, G. S., G. P. Zagaja, G. T. Bales, G. W. Chodak, and B. A. Contreras. "Saw Palmetto (Serenoa Repens) in Men With Lower Urinary Tract Symptoms: Effects on Urodynamic Parameters and Voiding Symptoms." *Urology* 51, no. 6 (June 1998): 1003–1007.

Gilbert, G. J. "Ginkgo Biloba." *Neurology* 48, no. 4 (April 1997): 1137.

Gionchetti, P., F. Rizzello, A. Venturi, and M. Campieri. "Probiotics in Infective Diarrhea and Inflammatory Bowel Diseases." *Journal of Gastroenterology and Hepatology* 15, no. 5 (May 2000): 489–493.

Godhwani, S., J. L. Godhwani, and D. S. Vyas. "Ocimum Sanctum: An Experimental Study Evaluating Its Anti-Inflammatory, Analgesic and Antipyretic Activity in Animals." *Journal of Ethnopharmacology* 21, no. 2 (November 1987): 153–163.

Gordon, M., B. Bihari, E. Goosby, et al. "A Placebo-Controlled Trial of the Immune Modulator, Lentinan, in HIV-Positive Patients: A Phase I/II Trial." *Journal of Medicine* 29, no. 5–6 (1998): 305–330.

Graham, I., L. E. Daly, H. M. Refsum, et al. "Plasma Homocysteine as a Risk Factor for Vascular Disease. The European Concerted Action Project." *Journal of the American Medical Association* 277, no. 22 (June 1997): 1775–1781.

Graham, S., R. Hellmann, J. Marshall, et al. "Nutritional Epidemiology of Postmenopausal Breast Cancer in Western New York." *American Journal of Epidemiology* 134, no. 6 (September 1991): 552–566.

Gunning, K. and P. Steele. "Echinacea for the Prevention of Upper Respiratory Tract Infections." *Journal of Family Practice* 48, no. 2 (February 1999): 93.

Halberstam, M., N. Cohen, P. Shlimovich, L. Rosetti, and H. Shamoon. "Oral Vanadyl Sulfate Improves Insulin Sensitivity in NIDDM but Not in Obese Nondiabetic Subjects." *Diabetes* 45, no. 5 (May 1996): 659–666.

Harvard Medical School, Health Publications Group. "A Special Report: High Blood Pressure." *Harvard Health Letter* (1990).

Hernandez, F., J. Illnait, and R. Mas. "Effect of Policosanol on Serum Lipids and Lipoproteins in Healthy Volunteers." *Current Therapeutic Research* 51 (1992): 568–575.

Hirano, T., M. Homma, and K. Oka. "Effects of Stinging Nettle Root Extracts and Their Steroidal Components on the Na+,K(+)-ATPase of the Benign Prostatic Hyperplasia." *Planta Medica* (Stuttgart) 60, no. 1 (February 1994): 30–33.

Hirasawa, M., N. Shouji, T. Neta, K. Fukushima, and K. Takada. "Three Kinds of Antibacterial Substances From Lentinus Edodes (Berk.) Sing. (Shiitake, an Edible Mushroom)." *International Journal of Antimicrobial Agents* (Amsterdam) 11, no. 2 (February 1999): 151–157.

Hirata, J. D., L. M. Swiersz, B. Zell, R. Small, and B. Ettinger. "Does Dong Quai Have Estrogenic Effects in Postmenopausal Women? A Double-Blind, Placebo-Controlled Trial." *Fertility and Sterility* 68, no. 6 (December 1997): 981–986.

Hirayama, K. and J. Rafter. "The Role of Probiotic Bacteria in Cancer Prevention." *Microbes and Infection* 2, no. 6 (May 2000): 681–686.

Hishida, I., H. Nanba, and H. Kuroda. "Antitumor Activity Exhibited by Orally Administered Extract From Fruit Body of *Grifola Frondosa* (Maitake)." *Chemical and Pharmaceutical Bulletin* (Tokyo) 36, no. 5 (May 1988): 1819–1827.

Hou, Y. D., G. L. Ma, S. H. Wu, Y. Y. Li, and H. T. Li. "Effect of *Radix Astragali Seu Hedysari* on the Interferon System." *Chinese Medical Journal* (English) (Beijing) 94, no. 1 (January 1981): 35–40.

Hryb, D. J., M. S. Khan, N. A. Romas, and W. Rosner. "The Effect of Extracts of the Roots of the Stinging Nettle (Urtica Dioica) on the Interaction of SHBG With Its Receptor on Human Prostatic Membranes." *Planta Medica* (Stuttgart) 61, no. 1 (February 1995): 31–32.

Hunter, D. J. and W. C. Willett. "Nutrition and Breast Cancer." *Cancer Causes Control* 7, no. 1 (January 1996): 56–68.

Imai, K. and K. Nakachi. "Cross Sectional Study of Effects of Drinking Green Tea on Cardiovascular and Liver Diseases."

British Medical Journal (London) 310, no. 6981 (March 1995): 693–696.

Ingram, D., K. Sanders, M. Kolybaba, and D. Lopez. "Case-Control Study of Phyto-Oestrogens and Breast Cancer." *Lancet* (London) 350, no. 9083 (November 1997): 990–994.

Jones, K. "Shiitake: A Major Medicinal Mushroom." *Alternative and Complementary Therapies* 4, no. 1 (February 1998): 53–59.

Kahn, R. S., H. G. Westenberg, W. M. Verhoeven, C. C. Gispen-de Wied, and W. D. Kamerbeek. "Effect of a Serotonin Precursor and Uptake Inhibitor in Anxiety Disorders; a Double-Blind Comparison of 5-Hydroxytryptophan, Clomipramine and Placebo." *International Clinical Psychopharmacology* (London) 2, no. 1 (January 1987): 33–45.

Kanowski, S., W. M. Herrmann, K. Stephan, W. Wierich, and R. Horr. "Proof of Efficacy of the *Ginkgo Biloba* Special Extract EGb 761 in Outpatients Suffering From Mild to Moderate Primary Degenerative Dementia of the Alzheimer Type or Multi-Infarct Dementia." *Pharmacopsychiatry* (Stuttgart) 29, no. 2 (March 1996): 47–56.

Kariya, Y., S. Watabe, K. Hashimoto, and K. Yoshida. "Occurrence of Chondroitin Sulfate E in Glycosaminoglycan Isolated From the Body Wall of Sea Cucumber Stichopus Japonicus." *Journal of Biological Chemistry* 265 (March 1990): 5081–5085.

Kawano, Y., H. Matsuoka, S. Takishita, and T. Omae. "Effects of Magnesium Supplementation in Hypertensive Patients: Assessment by Office, Home, and Ambulatory Blood Pressures." *Hypertension* 32, no. 2 (August 1998): 260–265.

Kelly, G. S. "The Role of Glucosamine Sulfate and Chondroitin Sulfates in the Treatment of Degenerative Joint Disease." *Alternative Medicine Review* 3, no. 1 (February 1998): 27–39.

Kelm, M. A., M. G. Nair, G. M. Strasburg, and D. L. DeWitt. "Antioxidant and Cyclooxygenase Inhibitory Phenolic Compounds From Ocimum Sanctum Linn." *Phytomedicine* (Stuttgart) 7, no. 1 (March 2000): 7–13.

Kennedy, A. R. "The Evidence for Soybean Products as Cancer Preventive Agents." *Journal of Nutrition* 125, no. 3 (March 1995): 733S–743S.

Khaw, K. and E. Barrett-Connor. "Dietary Potassium and Stroke Associated Mortality. A 12-Year Prospective Population Study." *New England Journal of Medicine* 316, no. 5 (January 1987): 235–240.

Kidd, P. M. "The Use of Mushroom Glucans and Proteoglycans in Cancer Treatment." *Alternative Medicine Review* 5, no. 1 (February 2000): 4–27.

Kleijnen, J. and P. Knipschild. "Ginkgo Biloba for Cerebral Insufficiency." *British Journal of Clinical Pharmacology* 34, no. 4 (October 1992): 352–358.

Klepser, T. and N. Nisly. "Astragalus as an Adjunctive Therapy in Immunocompromised Patients." *Integrative Medicine Alert* 2 (November 1999): 125–128.

Klippel, K. F., D. M. Hiltl, and B. Schipp. "A Multicentric, Placebo-Controlled, Double-Blind Clinical Trial of Beta-Sitosterol (Phytosterol) for the Treatment of Benign Prostatic Hyperplasia. German BPH-Phyto Study Group." *British Journal of Urology* 80, no. 3 (September 1997): 427–432.

Kono, S., K. Shinchi, N. Ikeda, F. Yanai, and K. Imanishi. "Green Tea Consumption and Serum Lipid Profiles: A Cross-Sectional Study in Northern Kyushu, Japan." *Preventive Medicine* 21, no. 4 (July 1992): 526–531.

Konrad, T., P. Vicini, K. Kusterer, et al. "Alpha Lipoic Acid Treatment Decreases Serum Lactate and Pyruvate Concentrations and Improves Glucose Effectiveness in Lean and Obese Patients With Type 2 Diabetes." *Diabetes Care* 22, no. 2 (February 1999): 280–287.

Kopp-Hoolihan, L. "Prophylactic and Therapeutic Uses of Probiotics: A Review." *Journal of the American Dietetic Association* 101, no. 2 (February 2001): 229–238.

Krishna, G. C., E. Miller, and S. Kapoor. "Increased Blood Pressure During Potassium Depletion in Normotensive Men." *New England Journal of Medicine* 320 (May 1989): 1177–1182.

Krzeski, T., M. Kazon, A. Borkowski, A. Witeska, and J. Kuczera. "Combined Extracts of Urtica Dioica and Pygeum Africanum in the Treatment of Benign Prostatic Hyperplasia: Double-Blind Comparison of Two Doses." *Clinical Therapeutics* 15, no. 6 (November–December 1993): 1011–1020.

Kulkarni, R. R., P. S. Patki, V. P. Jog, S. G. Gandage, and B. Patwardhan. "Treatment of Osteoarthritis With a Herbomineral Formulation: A Double-Blind, Placebo-Controlled, Cross-Over Study." *Journal of Ethnopharmacology* (Limerick) 33, no. 1–2 (May–June 1991): 91–95.

Kushi, L. H., A. R. Folsom, R. J. Prineas, et al. "Dietary Antioxidant Vitamins and Death From Coronary Heart Disease in Postmenopausal Women." *New England Journal of Medicine* 334, no. 18 (May 1996): 1156–1162.

Landrum, J. T., R. A. Bone, H. Joa, et al. "A One-Year Study of the Macular Pigment: The Effect of 140 Days of a Lutein Supplement." *Experimental Eye Research* 65, no. 1 (July 1997): 57–62.

Langsjoen, P., P. Langsjoen, R. Willis, and K. Folkers. "Treatment of Essential Hypertension With Coenzyme Q10." *Molecular Aspects of Medicine* (Oxford) 15 (1994): S265–S272.

Lansky, E. "Pomegranate Seed Oil Triggers Self-Destruct Mechanism in Breast Cancer Cells." Technion-Israel Institute of Technology. Paper presented in Madrid, June 2001.

Law, M. R., C. D. Frost, and N. J. Wald. "By How Much Does Dietary Salt Reduction Lower Blood Pressure? III—Analysis of Data From Trials of Salt Reduction." *British Medical Journal* 302, no. 6780 (April 1991): 819–924.

Le Bars, P. L., M. M. Katz, N. Berman, et al. "A Placebo-Controlled, Double-Blind, Randomized Trial of an Extract of *Ginkgo Biloba* for Dementia. North American EGb Study Group." *Journal of the American Medical Association* 278, no. 16 (October 1997): 1327–1332.

Lee, H. P., L. Gourley, S. W. Duffy, et al. "Dietary Effects on Breast-Cancer Risk in Singapore." *Lancet* (London) 337, no. 8751 (May 1991): 1197–1200.

Leicester, R. and R. H. Hunt. "Peppermint Oil to Reduce Colonic Spasm During Endoscopy." *Lancet* (London) 2, no. 8305 (October 1982): 989.

Lichius, J. J. and C. Muth. "The Inhibiting Effects of Urtica Dioica Root Extracts on Experimentally Induced Prostatic Hyperplasia in the Mouse." *Planta Medica* (Stuttgart) 63, no. 4 (August 1997): 307–310.

Lieberman, S. "A Review of the Effectiveness of *Cimicifuga Racemosa* (Black Cohosh) for the Symptoms of Menopause." *Journal of Women's Health* 7, no. 5 (June 1998): 525–529.

Loschen, G. and L. Ebeling. "Inhibition of Arachidonic Acid Cascade by Extract of Rye Pollen." *Arzneimittel-Forschung* (Germany) 41, no. 2 (February 1991): 162–167.

Lotz-Winter, H. "On the Pharmacology of Bromelain: An Update With Special Regard to Animal Studies on Dose-Dependent Effects." *Planta Medica* (Stuttgart) 56, no. 3 (June 1990): 249–253.

Lowe, F. C., K. Dreikorn, A. Borkowski, et al. "Review of Recent Placebo-Controlled Trials Utilizing Phytotherapeutic Agents for Treatment of BPH." *Prostate* 37, no. 3 (November 1998): 187–193.

Lyle, B. J., J. A. Mares-Perlman, B. E. Klein, R. Klein, and J. L. Greger. "Antioxidant Intake and Risk of Incident Age-Related Nuclear Cataracts in the Beaver Dam Eye Study." *American Journal of Epidemiology* 149, no. 8 (May 1999): 801–809.

MacDonald, R., A. Ishani, I. Rutks, and T. J. Wilt. "A Systematic Review of Cernilton for the Treatment of Benign Prostatic Hyperplasia." *British Journal of Urology International* (Oxford) 85, no. 7 (May 2000): 836–841.

Madar, Z., R. Abel, S. Samish, and J. Arad. "Glucose-Lowering Effect of Fenugreek in Non-Insulin Dependent Diabetics." *European Journal of Clinical Nutrition* (London) 42, no. 1 (January 1988): 51–54.

Maebashi, M., Y. Makino, Y. Furukawa, et al. "Therapeutic Evaluation of the Effect of Biotin on Hyperglycemia in Patients With

Non-Insulin Dependent Diabetes Mellitus." *Journal of Clinical Biochemistry and Nutrition* 14, no. 3 (1993): 211–218.

Marchioli, R. "Antioxidant Vitamins and Prevention of Cardiovascular Disease: Laboratory, Epidemiological and Clinical Trial Data." *Pharmacological Research* (London) 40, no. 3 (September 1999): 227–238.

Mares-Perlman, J. A., A. I. Fisher, R. Klein, et al. "Lutein and Zeaxanthin in the Diet and Serum and Their Relation to Age-Related Maculopathy in the Third National Health and Nutrition Examination Survey." *American Journal of Epidemiology* 153, no. 5 (March 2001): 424–432.

Martin, J. B. "Mortality Patterns Among Hypertensives by Reported Level of Caffeine Consumption." *Preventive Medicine* 17, no. 3 (May 1988): 310–320.

Mas, R., G. Castano, J. Illnait, et al. "Effects of Policosanol in Patients With Type II Hypercholesterolemia and Additional Coronary Risk Factors." *Clinical Pharmacology and Therapeutics* 65, no. 4 (April 1999): 439–447.

Mas, R., P. Rivas, J. E. Izquierdo, et al. "Pharmacoepidemiologic Study of Policosanol." *Current Therapeutic Research* 60, no. 8 (August 1999): 458–467.

Mathe, G., M. Hallard, C. H. Bourut, and E. Chenu. "A Pygeum Africanum Extract With So-Called Phyto-Estrogenic Action Markedly Reduces the Volume of True and Large Prostatic Hypertrophy." *Biomedicine and Pharmacotherapy* 49, no. 7–8 (1995): 341–343.

Mayell, M. "Maitake Extracts and Their Therapeutic Potential." *Alternative Medicine Review* 6, no. 1 (February 2001): 48–60.

McAlindon, T. E., M. P. LaValley, J. P. Gulin, and D. T. Felson. "Glucosamine and Chondroitin for Treatment of Osteoarthritis: A Systematic Quality Assessment and Meta-Analysis." *Journal of the American Medical Association* 283, no. 11 (March 2000): 1469–1475.

McCully, K. S. "Homocysteine and Vascular Disease." *Nature Medicine* 2, no. 4 (April 1996): 386–389.

Melchart, D., E. Walther, K. Linde, R. Brandmaier, and C. Lersch. "Echinacea Root Extracts for the Prevention of Upper Respiratory Tract Infections: A Double-Blind, Placebo-Controlled Randomized Trial." *Archives of Family Medicine* 7, no. 6 (November–December 1998): 541–545.

Menchini-Fabris, G. F., P. Giorgi, F. Andreini, et al. "New Perspectives on the Use of Pygeum Africanum in Prostato-Bladder Pathology." *Archivio Italiano Urologia, Nefrologia, e Andrologia* (Milano) 60, no. 3 (September 1988): 313–322.

Messina, M. J., V. Persky, K. D. Setchell, and S. Barnes. "Soy Intake and Cancer Risk: A Review of the *In Vitro* and *In Vivo* Data." *Nutrition and Cancer* 21, no. 2 (1994): 113–131.

Messina, M., S. Barnes, and K. D. Setchell. "Phyto-Oestrogens and Breast Cancer." *Lancet* (London) 350, no. 9083 (October 1997): 971–972.

Mizuno, M. "Anti-Tumor Polysaccharides From Mushrooms During Storage." *Biofactors* (Oxford) 12, no. 1–4 (2000): 275–281.

Mowrey, D. B. and D. E. Clayson. "Motion Sickness, Ginger, and Psychophysics." *Lancet* (London) 1, no. 8273 (March 1982): 655–657.

Muth, E. R., J. M. Laurent, and P. Jasper. "The Effect of Bilberry Nutritional Supplementation on Night Visual Acuity and Contrast Sensitivity." *Alternative Medicine Review* 5, no. 2 (April 2000): 164–173.

Nachtigall, L. B., L. La Grega, W. Lee, and R. Fenichel. "The Effects of Isoflavones Derived From Red Clover on Vasomotor Symptoms and Endometrial Thickness." In *Proceedings of the 9th International Menopause Society World Congress on the Menopause, Yokohama, Japan. October 17–21, 1999.* New York: Parthenon.

Nair, M. G. "MSU Study: Tart Cherries a Pain Killer." *Journal of Natural Products* (2000).

Nanba, H. "Antitumor Activity of Orally Administered 'D-Fraction' From Maitake Mushroom (Grifola Frondosa)." *Journal of Naturopathic Medicine* 4, no. 1 (1993): 10–15.

———. "Immunostimulant Activity In Vivo and Anti-HIV Activity In Vitro of 3 Branched b–1–6 Glucans Extracted From Maitake Mushrooms (*Grifola Frondosa*)." VIII International Conference on AIDS, Amsterdam, 1992.

Nanba, H. and H. Kuroda. "Antitumor Mechanisms of Orally Administered Shiitake Fruit Bodies." *Chemical and Pharmaceutical Bulletin* (Tokyo) 35, no. 6 (June 1987): 2459–2464.

Nanba, H., A. Hamaguchi, and H. Kuroda. "The Chemical Structure of an Antitumor Polysaccharide in Fruit Bodies of *Grifola Frondosa* (Maitake)." *Chemical and Pharmaceutical Bulletin* (Tokyo) 35, no. 3 (March 1987): 1162–1168.

Niewoehner, C. B., J. I. Allen, M. Boosalis, A. S. Levine, and J. E. Morley. "Role of Zinc Supplementation in Type II Diabetes Mellitus." *American Journal of Medicine* 81, no. 1 (July 1986): 63–68.

North American Menopause Society. "The Role of Isoflavones in Menopausal Health: Consensus of the North American Menopause Society." *Menopause* 7, no. 4 (July–August 2000): 215–229.

Ornish, D., S. E. Brown, L. W. Scherwitz, et al. "Can Lifestyle Changes Reverse Coronary Heart Disease? The Lifestyle Heart Trial." *Lancet* (London) 336, no. 8708 (July 1990): 129–133.

Otomo, E., J. Atarashi, G. Araki, et al. "Comparison of Vinpocetine With Ifenprodil Tartrate and Dihydroergotoxine Mesylate Treatment and Results of Long-Term Treatment With Vinpocetine." *Current Therapeutic Research* 37 (1985): 811–821.

Paolisso, G., S. Sgambto, G. Pizza, et al. "Improved Insulin Response and Action by Chronic Magnesium Administration in Aged NIDDM Subjects." *Diabetes Care* 12, no. 4 (April 1989): 265–269.

Patki, P. S., J. Singh, S. V. Gokhale, et al. "Efficacy of Potassium and Magnesium in Essential Hypertension: A Double-Blind, Placebo-Controlled, Crossover Study." *British Medical Journal* (London) 301, no. 6751 (September 1990): 521–523.

Persaud, S. J., H. Al-Majed, A Raman, and P. M. Jones. "Gymnema Sylvestre Stimulates Insulin Release In Vitro by Increased Membrane Permeability." *Journal of Endocrinology* 163, no. 2 (November 1999): 207–212.

Peterson, G. and S. Barnes. "Genistein Inhibits Both Estrogen and Growth Factor-Stimulated Proliferation of Human Breast Cancer Cells." *Cell Growth and Differentiation* 7, no. 10 (October 1996): 1345–1351.

Pittler, M. H. and E. Ernst. "Horse-Chestnut Seed Extract for Chronic Venous Insufficiency. A Criteria-Based Systematic Review." *Archives of Dermatology* 134, no. 11 (November 1998): 1356–1360.

Poldinger, W., B. Calanchini, and W. Schwarz. "A Functional-Dimensional Approach to Depression: Serotonin Deficiency As a Target Syndrome in a Comparison of 5-Hydroxytryptophan and Fluvoxamine." *Psychopathology* 24, no. 2 (1991): 53–81.

Polo, V., A. Saibene, and A. E. Pontiroli. "Nicotinamide Improves Insulin Secretion and Metabolic Control in Lean Type 2 Diabetic Patients With Secondary Failure to Sulphonylureas." *Acta Diabetologica Latina* (Berlin) 35, no. 1 (April 1998): 61–64.

Pons, P., A. Jimenez, M Rodriguez, et al. "Effects of Policosanol in Elderly Hypercholesterolemic Patients." *Current Therapeutic Research* 53, no. 3 (March 1993): 265–269.

Quella, S. K., C. L. Loprinzi, D. L. Barton, et al. "Evaluation of Soy Phytoestrogens for the Treatment of Hot Flashes in Breast Cancer Survivors: A North Central Cancer Treatment Group Trial." *Journal of Clinical Oncology* 18, no. 5 (March 2000): 1068–1074.

Qureshi, A. A., N. Qureshi, J. J. Wright, et al. "Lowering of Serum Cholesterol in Hypercholesterolemic Humans by Tocotrienols (Palmvitee)." *American Journal of Clinical Nutrition* 53, no. 4 (April 1991): 1021S–1026S.

Rajendran, S., P. D. Deepalakshmi, K. Parasakthy, H. Devaraj, and S. N. Devaraj. "Effects of Tincture of Crataegus on the LDL

Receptor Activity of Hepatic Plasma Membrane of Rats Fed an Atherogenic Diet." *Atherosclerosis* 123, no. 1–2 (June 1996): 235–241.

Rees, W., B. K. Evans, and J. Rhodes. "Treating Irritable Bowel Syndrome With Peppermint Oil." *British Medical Journal* (London) 2, no. 6194 (October 1979): 835–836.

Reginster, J. Y., R. Deroisy, L. C. Rovati, et al. "Long-Term Effects of Glucosamine Sulfate on Osteoarthritis Progression: A Randomised, Placebo-Controlled Clinical Trial." *Lancet* (London) 357, no. 9252 (January 2001): 251–256.

Reisin, E., R. Abel, M. Modan, et al. "Effect of Weight Loss Without Salt Restriction on the Reduction of Blood Pressure in Overweight Hypertensive Patients." *New England Journal of Medicine* 298, no. 1 (January 1978): 1–6.

Reljanovic, M., G. Reichel, K. Rett, et al. "Treatment of Diabetic Polyneuropathy With the Antioxidant Thioctic Acid (Alpha-Lipoic Acid): A Two Year Multicenter Randomized Double-Blind Placebo-Controlled Trial (ALADIN II). Alpha Lipoic Acid in Diabetic Neuropathy." *Free Radical Research* 31, no. 3 (September 1999): 171–179.

Rimm, E. B. and M. J. Stampfer. "Antioxidants for Vascular Disease." *Medical Clinics of North America* 84, no. 1 (January 2000): 239–249.

Rimm, E. B., M. J. Stampfer, A. Ascherio, et al. "Vitamin E Consumption and the Risk of Coronary Heart Disease in Men." *New England Journal of Medicine* 328, no. 20 (May 1993): 1450–1456.

Rimm, E. B., W. C. Willett, F. B. Hu, et al. "Folate and Vitamin B6 From Diet and Supplements in Relation to Risk of Coronary Heart Disease Among Women." *Journal of the American Medical Association* 279, no. 5 (February 1998): 359–364.

Rosenberg, I. H. and J. W. Miller. "Nutritional Factors in Physical and Cognitive Functions of Elderly People." *American Journal of Clinical Nutrition* 55, no. 6 (June 1992): 1237S–1243S.

Sacks, F. M. "Dietary Fats and Blood Pressure: A Critical Review of
     the Evidence." *Nutrition Reviews* 47, no. 10 (October 1989):
     291–300.

Sano, M., Y. Takahashi, K. Shimoi, et al. "Effect of Tea (Camellia
     Sinensis L.) on Lipid Peroxidation in Rat Liver and Kidney: A
     Comparison of Green and Black Tea Feeding." *Biological and
     Pharmaceutical Bulletin* (Tokyo) 18, no. 7 (July 1995): 1006–1008.

Santos, M. S., S. N. Meydani, L. Leka, et al. "Natural Killer Cell
     Activity in Elderly Men Is Enhanced by Beta-Carotene
     Supplementation." *American Journal of Clinical Nutrition* 64,
     no. 5 (November 1996): 772–777.

Schelber, M. D. and R. W. Rebar. "Isoflavones and Postmenopausal
     Bone Health: A Viable Alternative to Estrogen Therapy?"
     Menopause 6, no. 3 (Fall 1999): 233–241.

Seddon, J. M., U. A. Ajani, R. D. Sperduto, et al. "Dietary Carotenoids,
     Vitamins A, C, and E, and Advanced Age-Related Macular
     Degeneration. Eye Disease Case-Control Study Group."
     Journal of the American Medical Association 272, no. 18
     (November 1994): 1413–1420.

Segars, L. W. "Saw Palmetto Extracts for Benign Prostatic
     Hyperplasia." *Journal of Family Practice* 48, no. 2 (February
     1999): 88–89.

Selhub, J., P. F. Jacques, P. W. Wilson, D. Rush, and I. H. Rosenberg.
     "Vitamin Status and Intake as Primary Determinants of
     Homocysteinemia in an Elderly Population." *Journal of the
     American Medical Association* 270, no. 22 (December 1993):
     2693–2698.

Semba, R. D. "Vitamin A, Immunity, and Infection." *Clinical Infectious
     Diseases* 19, no. 3 (September 1994): 489–499.

Serafini, M., A. Ghiselli, and A. Ferro-Luzzi. "In Vivo Antioxidant
     Effect of Green and Black Tea in Man." *European Journal of
     Clinical Nutrition* (London) 50, no. 1 (January 1996): 28–32.

Shanmugasundaram, E. R., G. Rajeswari, K. Baskaran, et al. "Use
     of Gymnema Sylvestre Leaf Extract in the Control of Blood
     Glucose in Insulin-Dependent Diabetes Mellitus." *Journal*

of Ethnopharmacology (Limerick) 30, no. 3 (October 1990): 281–294.

Sharma, R. D., T. C. Raghuram, and N. S. Rao. "Effect of Fenugreek Seeds on Blood Glucose and Serum Lipids in Type 1 Diabetes." *European Journal of Clinical Nutrition* (London) 44, no. 4 (April 1990): 301–306.

Simon, J. A. and E. S. Hudes. "Serum Ascorbic Acid and Other Correlates of Self-Reported Cataract Among Older Americans." *Journal of Clinical Epidemiology* (Oxford) 52, no. 12 (December 1999): 207–211.

Sinatra, S. T. "Coenzyme Q10: A Vital Therapeutic Nutrient for the Heart With Special Application in Congestive Heart Failure." *Connecticut Medicine* 61, no. 11 (November 1997): 707–711.

Singh, S., D. K. Majumdar, and H. M. Rehan. "Evaluation of Anti-Inflammatory Potential of Fixed Oil of Ocimum Sanctum (Holybasil) and Its Possible Mechanism of Action." *Journal of Ethnopharmacology* (Limerick) 54, no. 1 (October 1996): 19–26.

Stensvold, I., A. Tverdal, K. Solvoll, and O. P. Foss. "Tea Consumption. Relationship to Cholesterol, Blood Pressure, and Coronary and Total Mortality." *Preventive Medicine* 21, no. 4 (July 1992): 546–553.

Stoll, B. A. "Eating to Beat Breast Cancer: Potential Role for Soy Supplements." *Annals of Oncology* (Dordrecht) 8, no. 3 (March 1997): 223–225.

Stusser, R., J. Batista, R. Padron, F. Sosa, and O. Pereztol. "Long-Term Therapy With Policosanol Improves Treadmill Exercise-ECG Testing Performance of Coronary Heart Disease Patients." *International Journal of Clinical Pharmacology and Therapeutics* (Munchen) 36, no. 9 (September 1998): 469–473.

Sun, Q. Q., S. S. Xu, J. L. Pan, H. M. Guo, and W. Q. Cao. "Huperzine-A Capsules Enhance Memory and Learning Performance in 34 Pairs of Matched Adolescent Students." *Zhongguo Yao Li Xue Bao* (Beijing) 20, no. 7 (July 1999): 601–603.

Sun, Y., E. M. Hersh, M. Talpaz, et al. "Immune Restoration and/ or Augmentation of Local Graft Versus Host Reaction by Traditional Chinese Medicinal Herbs." *Cancer* 52, no. 1 (July 1983): 70–73.

Taguchi, I. "Clinical Efficacy of Lentinan on Patients With Stomach Cancer: End Point Results of a Four-Year Follow-Up Survey." *Cancer Detection and Prevention.* Supplement 1 (1987): 333–349.

Taussig, S. J. and S. Batkin. "Bromelain, the Enzyme Complex of Pineapple (Ananas Comosus) and Its Clinical Application. An Update." *Journal of Ethnopharmacology* 22, no. 2 (February– March 1988): 191–203.

Taylor, M. "Alternatives to Hormone Replacement Therapy." *Comprehensive Therapy* 23 (1997): 514–532.

Teikari, J. M., J. Virtamo, M. Rautalahti, et al. "Long-Term Supplementation With Alpha-Tocopherol and Beta-Carotene and Age-Related Cataract." *Acta Ophthalmologica Scandinavica* (Hvidovre) 75, no. 6 (December 1997): 634–640.

Thacker, H. L. and D. L. Booher. "Management of Perimenopause: Focus on Alternative Therapies." *Cleveland Clinic Journal of Medicine* 66, no. 4 (April 1999): 213–218.

Thomas, S. R., J. Neuzil, and R. Stocker. "Inhibition of LDL Oxidation by Ubiquinol-10. A Protective Mechanism for Coenzyme Q10 in Atherogenesis?" *Molecular Aspects of Medicine* (Oxford) 18, supplement (1997): 85–103.

Tomeo, A. C., M. Geller, T. R. Watkins, A. Gapor, and M. L. Bierenbaum. "Antioxidant Effects of Tocotrienols in Patients With Hyperlipidemia and Carotid Stenosis." *Lipids* 30, no. 12 (December 1995): 1179–1183.

Van Dongen, M. C., E. van Rossum, A. G. Kessels, H. J. Sielhorst, and P. G. Knipschild. "The Efficacy of Ginkgo for Elderly People With Dementia and Age-Associated Memory Impairment: New Results of a Randomized Clinical Trial." *Journal of the American Geriatrics Society* 48, no. 10 (October 2000): 1183–1194.

Ved, H. S., M. L. Koenig, J. R. Dave, and B. P. Doctor. "Huperzine A, a Potential Therapeutic Agent for Dementia, Reduces

Neuronal Cell Death Caused by Glutamate." *Neuroreport* (Oxford) 8, no. 4 (March 1997): 963–968.

Venter, C. S., H. S. Kruger, H. H. Vorster, et al. "The Effects of Dietary Fiber Component Konjac-Glucomannan on Serum Cholesterol Levels of Hypercholesterolemic Subjects." *Hum Nutr Food Sci Nutr* 41 (1987): 55–61.

Vieira, R. P., C. Pedrosa, and P. A. Mourao. "Extensive Heterogeneity of Proteoglycans Bearing Fucose-Branched Chondroitin Sulfate Extracted From the Connective Tissue of Sea Cucumber." *Biochemistry* 32, no. 9 (March 1993): 2254–2262.

Vuksan, V., D. J. Jenkins, P. Spadafora, et al. "Konjac-Mannan (Glucomannan) Improves Glycemia and Other Associated Risk Factors for Coronary Heart Disease in Type 2 Diabetes. A Randomized Controlled Metabolic Trial." *Diabetes Care* 22, no. 6 (June 1999): 913–919.

Wang, H., M. G. Nair, G. M. Strasburg, A. M. Borren, and J. I. Gray. "Novel Antioxidant Compounds From Tart Cherries (Prunus Cerasus)." *Journal of Natural Products* 62, no. 1 (January 1999): 86–88.

Warnecke, G. "Influencing Menopausal Symptoms With a Phytotherapeutic Agent: Successful Therapy With *Cimicifuga* Mono-Extract." *Die Medizinische Welt* (Stuttgart) 36 (1985): 871–874.

Weikl, A., K. D. Assmus, A. Neukum-Schmidt, et al. "Crataegus Special Extract WS 1442. Assessment of Objective Effectiveness in Patients With Heart Failure." *Fortschritte Der Medizin* (Munich) 114, no. 24 (August 1996): 291–296.

Whelton, P. K., L. J. Appel, M. A. Espeland, et al. "Sodium Reduction and Weight Loss in the Treatment of Hypertension in Older Persons: A Randomized Controlled Trial of Nonpharmacologic Interventions in the Elderly (TONE). TONE Collaborative Research Group." *Journal of the American Medical Association* 279, no. 11 (March 1998): 839–846.

Wilt, T. J., A. Ishani, G. Stark, et al. "Saw Palmetto Extracts for Treatment of Benign Prostatic Hyperplasia: A Systematic

Review." *Journal of the American Medical Association* 280, no. 18 (November 1998): 1604–1609.

Wilt, T. J., R. MacDonald, and A. Ishani. "Beta-Sitosterol for the Treatment of Benign Prostatic Hyperplasia: A Systematic Review." *British Journal of Urology International* (Oxford) 83, no. 9 (June 1999): 976–983.

Wolf, A., C. Zalpour, G. Theilmeier, et al. "Dietary L-Arginine Supplementation Normalizes Platelet Aggregation in Hypercholesterolemic Humans." *Journal of the American College of Cardiology* 29, no. 3 (March 1997): 479–485.

Xu, S. S., Z. X. Gao, Z. Weng, et al. "Efficacy of Tablet Huperzine-A on Memory, Cognition, and Behavior in Alzheimer's Disease." *Zhongguo Yao Li Xue Bao* (Beijing) 16, no. 5 (September 1995): 391–395.

Yamada, Y., H. Nanba, and H. Kuroda. "Antitumor Effect of Orally Administered Extracts From Fruit Body of *Grifola Frondosa* (Maitake)." *Chemical and Pharmaceutical Bulletin* (Tokyo) 38 (1990): 790–796.

Zakay-Rones, Z., N. Varsano, M. Zlotnik, et al. "Inhibition of Several Strains of Influenza Virus In Vitro and Reduction of Symptoms by an Elderberry Extract (Sambucus Nigra L.) During an Outbreak of Influenza B Panama." *Journal of Alternative and Complementary Medicine* 1, no. 4 (Winter 1995): 361–369.

Zhang, S., D. J. Hunter, M. R. Forman, et al. "Dietary Carotenoids and Vitamins A, C, and E and Risk of Breast Cancer." *Journal of the National Cancer Institute* 91, no. 6 (March 1999): 547–556.

Zhang, X., J. Z. Ouyang, Y. S. Zhang, et al. "Effect of the Extracts of Pumpkin Seeds on the Urodynamics of Rabbits: An Experimental Study." *Journal of Tongji Medical University* (Wuhan) 14, no. 4 (1994): 235–238.

Zheng, Z., D. Liu, C. Song, C. Cheng, and Z. Hu. "Studies on Chemical Constituents and Immunological Function Activity of Hairy Root of Astragalus Membranaceus." *Chinese Journal of Biotechnology* (New York) 14, no. 2 (1998): 93–97.

INDEX

CONNECT WITH US!

CHARISMA HOUSE

(Spiritual Growth)

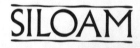

Facebook.com/CharismaHouse

@CharismaHouse

Instagram.com/CharismaHouse

SILOAM

(Health)

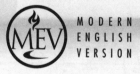

Pinterest.com/CharismaHouse

MEV MODERN ENGLISH VERSION

(Bible)

www.mevbible.com